Preface

Within this book are twelve scripts designed to excite and arouse a partner with hypnotic, erotic language.

If you use them, please ensure you are clear about the contents of the scripts you use, and acquire informed, enthusiastic consent from the person you hypnotize. The scripts generally assume that consent has been given and do not include that element of negotiation and pre-talk that is necessary before a hypnosis session.

It is important to discuss your intentions, and what will happen. Not only will that make for a happier subject, it will also help them to trust you, which will make the hypnosis more effective.

In addition, ensure to take some time for aftercare once you finish. Ask your subject how they felt during the session. Most of all, make sure they felt safe in trance.

These scripts are focused on a dominant/submissive dynamic, so please do bear in mind that they are written from the perspective of a dominant hypnotizing someone who is submissive to them. Some are gender-neutral, others are focused on a male subject, but you can quite easily change the named body parts to suit the gender of your subject.

There are several moments in these scripts where a non-verbal sound effect is required, such as snapping your fingers. When these occur, you will see the sound effect described in bracketed italicized text, like this:

(snap your fingers)

I hope you, and your subject, enjoy these scripts and have fun exploring the wonderful world of erotic hypnosis.

X

Calia

Disclaimer

Hypnosis, despite the media interpretation, is not mind control. It requires the trust, and consent of all participants to be effective. It is also not sleep; it is a state of intense focus. Your goal with these scripts is not to put your partner to sleep, but to have them focus so intently that they become suggestible, and open to ideas and fantasies that they enjoy in a way that allows them to drop their inhibitions and embrace the scene.

When I write erotic hypnosis, I write it based on just that, scenes. In a BDSM sense, a scene is a moment in time. An agreed-upon shared experience involving whatever fantasy the participants like, with all necessary work done to ensure safety. Once the scene ends, so does the fantasy, we are no longer Mistress and slave, or Master and Sub, we are once more peers, equals, friends or lovers.

With that in mind, please remember, everything you read is for fantasy only. Using hypnosis demands you take the time to acquire consent from your partner, and to ensure they are happy and comfortable before, during, and after your sessions and scenes. Suggestions that go beyond trance, into post-hypnotic suggestion, should be used with consent and with regard to reality. Nothing here should be used in a way that violates legal, ethical, moral, or personal boundaries.

Hypnosis is a tool to increase enjoyment of domination, submission, and erotic play. Much like a paddle used to spank someone, you should know the limits of the subject, and be keenly aware of when they are and are not enjoying themselves. Take care to look out for body language or expressions that indicate discomfort, and ensure they feel comfortable throughout any session.

If you would like to learn more about how to ensure your partner is enjoying the experience, the book Mindplay by Mark Wiseman is a fabulous resource, which will absolutely improve your experiences with these scripts, should you read it.

SCRIPTS

Click Trigger

This script is designed to give your subject a trigger, to return to a state of trance and feel a jolt of pleasure as they do. It's a nice, simple way to demonstrate your power and a trigger you can use in future sessions to induce trance more quickly and make sure your subject is suitably excited for the experience.

I want you to start by taking a long, deep breath. Don't worry about holding it, don't worry about when you release. Just a long, deep breath in and out, in your own time.

Keep doing that as you listen to me and feel the air moving into your body and back out, slowly, and gently filling your lungs, then emptying them. The gentle swell of your chest and the subtle scents in the air around you.

It's very easy to do, to just breathe in and out. You can keep doing it as you listen even if we talk about something else.

You don't have to think about it, all you have to do is breathe. Rhythmically, slowly, and gently.

As you breathe in and out, you begin to feel relaxed. As the air moves through you, you let a pleasant feeling of relaxation and calm wash over you.

That's right. It starts at your feet. You feel your toes, wiggle them a little, but with each breath, they get more relaxed, heavier. It's a nice feeling, a soft, warm feeling.

It moves up your ankles into your legs next. Everything just getting heavy and limp as you breathe softly and slowly. It's a wonderful feeling, isn't it? Nod your head yes.

Good, you can keep breathing slowly now, letting your thoughts drift to whatever you like, just listen to my voice, and breathe, that's all you need to do as the soft warmth moves into your thighs now.

You feel that warm sensation as it relaxes your legs, from your waist down. You can just gently nod yes if you agree. Do you feel it, the relaxation that has fallen over you?

Good, keep breathing for me, that's right. You just listen and breathe and relax. You start to notice your stomach now, that gentle glow spreading through your torso, a warmth moving through you, up into your chest. It's pleasant, safe and oh so relaxing, isn't it?

Of course it is, it feels good to let yourself relax, to just slow down your breathing and let your body sink down until you could barely move, not that you want to.

That heavy, warm feeling moves up your back into your neck and shoulders, like a gentle massage. You breathe in and out and your muscles relax and unwind, don't they?

That's right, you can feel your arms now, your hands, they seem to have lost any energy and you just let them fall limp at your sides as your mind fills with my relaxing, soothing words.

Now as that warmth moves up your neck, you can just switch off your thoughts, your cares. You only listen and breathe as you empty your mind and let yourself absorb what I say. Let yourself get lost in the warmth and comfort of my voice.

That's it, let your mind open to my words, to my calming, warm words. It feels good to switch off your thoughts and let mine in, to switch off from the world, like someone moving their finger toward the switch on a lamp, ready to click and put it out.

You want me to flick that switch for you, to click and turn off all those thoughts, all those things from the outside world that intrude on us here, where we feel safe and warm and wonderful, don't you?

Yes, very good. So calm and relaxed for me, so ready to switch off, to drop down into a state of sleep for me.

I'm going to count from ten to one, and with each number I will get a little closer to the switch, the one that will shut off your mind and leave it empty of anything but my words. Are you ready?

That's right, ten.

Feeling yourself falling into a blissfully relaxed place.

Nine.

Seeing my hand, my fingers, moving toward the switch.

Eight.

Ready to fall deep for me.

Seven.

Breathing slowly in and out.

Six.

Letting your body stay limp, relaxed, and comfortable.

Five.

Feeling my words pull you down deeper.

Four.

Seeing the switch in your mind, and my hand drawing nearer.

Three.

Feeling warm, wonderfully relaxed and oh so sleepy.

Two.

Almost there, almost in a state of calm, warm, trance.

One.

(Snap your fingers)

You feel the thoughts slip from your mind as I flick the switch and shut off your brain. No more thoughts, no more worries. You breathe and you listen. You know the click brought you down to this state and you know it feels wonderful.

You are relaxed all over. Your entire body feels warm and comfortable. It is a wonderful, pleasurable feeling. You find yourself enjoying the heaviness of your body, the emptiness of your mind.

You realise that you are glad I took you down into this state. You breathe in and out slowly and feel happy to be in my power, in my trance.

You belong here.

And you can get lost in that feeling, as you feel the warmth of my voice wrapping around your empty mind.

That's right, the softness of my voice makes your mind fill with thoughts and desires to fall deeper under my power. You enjoy that feeling, it feels good. It feels right.

I want you to breathe in and out for me again, even slower than before. Falling even deeper now, into my relaxing trance. Even deeper into my power.

Your mind is empty, your thoughts are my words. You love this feeling.

That's right, you nod your head yes because you know that I'm right. You love to relax and shut off your mind for me.

You feel so good in this sleepy, drowsy state.

Warm, comfortable and calm.

But other feelings drift around in your mind. Your thoughts are gone, but emotions, desires, they remain. The warmth that fills your body is not only calming, but also gives you a little

pleasure, and you feel it more now, feel it growing inside you.

It's a lovely feeling, a gentle, calm pleasure. The pleasure of simply switching off and letting me take control.

It makes you feel very good, and the more I speak, the better it feels. The more you open yourself up to me and listen, the better it feels.

Isn't that right?

Good, keep listening and breathing slowly as you feel that pleasure grow even more. You feel the tingle of arousal creeping through your body.

It's like electricity on your skin. You feel it on your right arm, a tingling, teasing sensation. Now on your left. Like an invisible fingernail scraping gently across the skin.

Now you feel it on the back of your neck, making the hairs stand on end. It's just a tingle, a jolt of sensation, but you enjoy it, and now you know that in this state of trance that I can give it to you.

You know that being here with me, in a deep, pleasurable trance, is something you are coming to really enjoy.

Now we're going to take you even deeper. I'm going to teach you a little trigger that will help bring you back to this pleasant state, and increase the pleasure you feel.

You know that the click brought you here, the click of a switch, like the click of my fingernails… like this:

(*Snap your fingers*)

And when you hear that click, you will feel yourself being pulled back to this state, pulled back into my power.

Not only that, every time you hear the (*Snap your fingers*)

you will feel that jolt of pleasure, as if my fingernail is scraping along the back of your neck.

Each (*Snap your fingers*) will bring you deeper, take you closer to my trance until you can no longer resist, and fall completely, feeling the switch in your mind go off, and your thoughts vanish into nothing.

That jolt of pleasure that my (*Snap your fingers*) brings will remind you of the pleasurable sensation of being in my power, and push you down, make you relax and give in to the desire to just let go of thought and drift into trance for me.

And I want you to take that with you today, take that feeling and that memory. I want you to remember for me, that my (*Snap your fingers*) pulls you into my trance and sends a jolt of pleasure through your body.

And I want you to remember how good it felt to fall into my power, but only in your subconscious mind. Your conscious mind will only have a vague, fuzzy recollection that you enjoyed listening to me and my voice, and you want to do so again.

Now, in a moment I will wake you, and you will go back to the world with all your thoughts intact, but with just that one new one – my (*Snap your fingers*) takes you down into trance with a jolt of pleasure.

So if you are ready, I will count up from one to five, and at five you will be fully awake and alert.

One.

Feel the heaviness start to leave your body.

Two.

Thoughts swimming back into your mind.

Three.

Eyes blinking, toes wiggling, feeling returns.

Four.

Aware of the world around you and feeling loose and light.

And five.

Fully awake now, feeling alert and refreshed.

Obedience is Pleasure

This script is designed to increase the arousal of your subject when they follow your commands. This script is an ideal early one to use, as it can increase the potential pleasure of later sessions with a simple reminder that it feels quite nice to follow the orders of your hypnotist. This also includes an amnesia trigger, your subject should forget most of what they heard, leaving them with just one thing – the knowledge that obedience is pleasure.

Let's begin, shall we?

Yes, you want to begin, don't you? Begin to rest your body. Begin to feel your arms and legs weaken and soften and your breathing slow.

Begin to notice the world around you drifting away, like its fading, no longer important.

Begin to feel your toes and your fingers loosen. Begin to feel your eyelids flutter as they grow heavier.

It's nice to feel this way, to just relax and rest your body.

You enjoy this feeling, you enjoy the beginning of a nice, relaxing trance. The moments before you drop deep, when you still notice the little things around you, but realise they don't matter.

You know that at the beginning, you are awake, but not really, not fully. You feel the urge to just listen and let go and that feels so nice.

That's right, it feels so nice to just listen to me and begin to forget the world around you as you fall down. Down into a gentle state of relaxation. A peaceful, calming place.

Let me be your guide from the beginning, let me take you down, pull you with me into the depths of a trance.

You know how nice that feels already because as you listen to my words you can feel the beginning melting into the middle and the world melting into nothing. It's like being pulled down into the depths of a warm bath or a blue-green sea.

You just want to slide back, your shoulders going limp, and relax.

Mmm, yes that feels so nice.

Just let yourself rest and relax as you listen to my words. You might still notice the sounds of the place where you are sitting, but you realise they are very far away. You're drifting down underwater, under my trance, and those sounds are getting further from you with every word I say.

Every word I say taking you deeper into the warm depths of trance, every word making the world disappear a little more.

You want to keep falling with me, to keep diving down ever deeper, and all you have to do is listen to my words.

All you have to do is follow me and listen. It's so very, very easy.

That's right, let go, let the world go and fall down deeper and deeper with me, for me, into this state of blissful relaxation.

Your body is relaxed, limp, weightless. Your mind is filled with my words, no room for anything else. Just falling, drifting down and down and down.

My words are like that warm water, wrapping you up, covering you, making you feel as though you're floating.

You enjoy that feeling, that feeling of weight vanishing, the pressure lifting from you. There is nothing but my words, my warm, soft words that take you down. You fall, your worries and cares stay up on the surface.

Here in this warm, wonderful trance, you simply listen and let go, listen and fall deeper. Leave everything else behind and follow my words. My words are all you need, all you want.

That's right, now you find yourself falling slowly down into warm, deep waters with me. You are weightless, my words are pulling you.

I am going to count from ten to one, and with each number you will find yourself falling even deeper into the dark depths of relaxation and trance, until I reach one, and when I do, the surface will be out of sight as you shut your eyes and fall fully into trance.

Feeling yourself falling now, leaving the surface and the waking world behind.

Ten.

Your weightless body drifts down with every word I say.

Nine.

Mind emptying of thought and filling with my words.

Eight.

Safe and calm in the warm depths of my voice.

Seven.

Falling down deeper into trance with me.

Six.

Your body feels warm and calm, totally relaxed.

Five.

Your mind is clear of thought and open to new ideas.

Four.

You are ready to embrace the depths of trance.

Three.

Light fades, your eyes flicker closed if they are still open.

Two.

The sounds of the outside world vanish, only my words remain.

One.

Totally entranced, deep down, deeply asleep. In the dark depths of trance.

You feel so warm, so safe and so light here. This perfect, pleasurable place of total calm. Your body is loose, limp and light. Your mind is empty of thought, only my words are needed here.

You followed my words down, and now my words will guide you further.

I will guide you toward a new mindset, a new way of thinking, that will help you feel calm and relaxed always.

But to get there, I need you to trust me. I need you to nod your head as you realise that this is what you want. You want to trust me, and to follow me.

That's it, feel your head nod in agreement. You want to feel relaxed, and I can make sure you do, whether deep in trance or in the waking world which feels so, so far away now.

And you can go even deeper. You just have to follow me. I want you to follow me now and imagine a cave under the water. You are drifting toward it. Inside it is bright, and you can only see white.

Picture it, in your mind's eye, a cave in the dark depths, filled with white light. As you drift closer, pulled by my words, details appear. It is a place you remember, a place that has always made you feel happy.

You notice things about it from deep in your memories, objects, decorations, that draw you back to that happy place as you are drawn in.

That place is one of great calm for you, and you will soon be there, with my words the soft blanket wrapping you in warmth, the gentle hand guiding you to happiness.

You realise that following me makes you happy. Brings you happiness.

You know that if you follow my words, you will feel good.

That makes so much sense to you.

That's right.

As you drift into that place of happiness, you fall ever deeper into trance and know that when you follow me, listen to me, you feel happy. You feel the pleasurable warmth that can only come from listening to me, and following my words.

Now so close to the entrance to the cave, you will be there in moments, guided by my words. Once you cross the threshold you will fall into an even deeper state of trance. A place so deep that your mind will be totally empty, your body will be totally relaxed, and you will be ready to listen to my words and let them fill your mind.

Entering the cave in five

Seeing that happy place in your mind.

Four.

Knowing that I can bring you here.

Three.

Knowing that I can bring you happiness.

Two.

Allowing my words to fill your mind and empty it of thought.

One.

Enter it now, that place that makes you so happy. Guided by my words, my voice.

You love it here, it is the warmest, most pleasurable place you know.

And I brought you here.

My trance, my words, all brought you happiness.

You feel a smile creep across your lips as you recognise what I have done for you.

And you start to understand that when you follow me, happiness is the result.

When you listen to me, it makes you feel so good.

When you simply let go and let me take control, you are happy.

Listening to me is pleasure itself. It makes you feel good, makes you feel safe, makes you feel warm and soft and wonderful.

All you have to do is let your thoughts go, and let mine in. Let my words guide you.

Obey my words, and pleasure and happiness will be yours.

Obeying me is so easy, my voice in your ear is your guide. Simply listen and obey.

That's all you have to do, listen and obey.

And obedience is pleasure, because when you obey and follow me, I take you to the happy places in your mind.

Obedience is pleasure because I make you feel weightless and wonderful.

Obedience is pleasure, remember that.

You are so deep in trance that you won't remember anything else, but your mind will hold onto that phrase, that thought, that idea.

Obedience is pleasure.

That's right.

Obedience is pleasure.

And all you have to do, to feel happy and good and warm, is to follow and obey me.

It's so easy. So simple.

You can forget everything else, forget everything else but deep in your subconscious mind, you know that obedience is pleasure and obeying me is so easy, and makes you feel so good.

In fact, when you obey me, you will smile and feel the same warmth you feel in that happy place deep in the depths of trance. You will feel so good when you obey me.

That's all you need to remember, that obeying me makes you feel good, makes you smile, makes you happy.

Obedience is pleasure.

And now I'm going to draw you up from the depths with me, bring you back to the surface. We went down so far that I need to count from one to ten to bring us back up.

You will remember that obedience is pleasure, but your mind will let the details disappear as you rise up while I count from one.

Feeling your body moving up with me, with my words.

Two.

Your thoughts starting to return, slowly.

Three.

Sounds of the outside world coming back from afar.

Four.

Your body moves up and your limbs start to move a little.

Five.

Seeing the light of the surface now as you open your eyes

Six.

Mind clearing, forgetting everything but obedience is pleasure.

Seven.

Body warm and refreshed, feeling so good.

Eight.

Eyelids blinking, shake your shoulders out.

Nine.

Wonderfully calm, but alert and almost awake.

Ten.

Fully awake, at the surface now, feeling a sense of incredible peace and calm.

You had a wonderful relaxing experience, but now it's time to go back to the waking world. I'm so glad we could share this time together. I would love if you could do one small thing for me, now you are awake, just tell me, who do you obey?

Silken Strings

In this script, your subject experiences two, shall we say, 'tropey' induction techniques. One is asking them to raise a hand as if you are controlling it, the other, descending a staircase. They're somewhat cliché but remain effective and particularly potent if your subject is aware of such tropes. The rest of the script is about making them feel as if they are your puppet, guided by your silken strings.

I want you to do something very simple for me. It will be easy, just a small request.

I want you to think about your right hand.

It might sound a little odd, to think about your right hand. It's always there, a constant companion. You don't usually think about it. Your hand just… is.

But now, I want you to feel it. Feel the blood moving through your veins, the slight twitch of your muscles, the curl of your fingers. You notice the weight of it, the way it sits by your side or by your chair or on your desk. Its heavy, you must think about lifting it.

You feel that don't you? You feel your hand growing heavier as you think about it. A strange, unexpected sensation, like its falling down, pulled by an unseen force.

That's ok, that's what you should feel, and even if you don't, just thinking about your hand is ok, just focus on it.

Now I want you to imagine for me, imagine that hand is being tied up in string. Soft, gentle loops wrapping around it. They feel nice, secure, and not too tight. The string wraps around your hand several times, going around your palm and over the back, then looping around again.

You feel it loop again and again, building up strong strands of string, but your fingers and thumb are free to move still. You are not restrained, not restricted, just feeling strand after strand of string around your right hand.

You can almost picture it; the string is white and slightly transparent. It wraps your hand up then the rest shoots straight up, toward the ceiling, off to somewhere unseen far above.

You do not need to worry about where the string leads, you only need to remember that your hand is tied and the string tying it vanishes up above you.

It is important that you remember that as you think about your hand, just as I asked you to.

You've been very patient as I explained all the details I wanted you to consider. I am pleased with how you are doing.

You have done such a good job thinking about your right hand, that naturally, your attention shifts to your left. You lose a little focus and that's ok. Your left hand is lighter, it wants to move, to float upward.

You don't remember it being lighter than your right hand, but now that you think about it deeply, it is. It is almost weightless. You start to feel it rise up, almost of its own accord. You are not doing anything to make this happen.

That's right, your left hand rises slowly into the air until it stops, and just hangs limply above you.

Then you feel it, feel the string again, just like your right hand. You realise that your left hand is also wrapped in the fine layers of string, and those strings loop together tightly, but not too tightly, and lead to a line of string that goes up, up, up into the air above you.

You feel a gentle tug on that string and your hand bounces upward, then goes back to where it stopped before, hanging.

Your hand is suspended on a string. Your right hand now, just like the left, feels the pull of the string. The gentle but insistent tug from above. Your right hand begins to rise and slowly, slowly it moves up.

The feeling is strange, you are not fighting it, just allowing your hands to be pulled up by the strings. Your right hand is soon level with your left, floating, limp and lifeless.

You realise that you are being pulled up by an unseen force as you sit or lie down and relax.

Relax and let the strings pull on you. Let them hold your hands up where they are, and now feel them start to lower your hands down.

Feel them letting your hands fall slowly back to a resting position.

As I count down from five to one, your hands will slowly move back to where they started, and once they hit the surface beneath them, whether it is a bed, an armrest or even your own body, you will slip into a deep trance.

Five.

Feeling the strings as they lower your hands down gently.

Four.

Letting yourself relax and give up control of your body.

Three.

Feeling the strings around your hands, letting them control your movement.

Two.

Almost down now, almost in a trance for me.

And one.

Your hands are at rest, and so are you. You are in a gentle, relaxing trance. Your hands are still wrapped up in string, and as you relax, you feel the same string wrapping your mind up. Like silk, weaving its way into your brain and slowing you down.

You feel the pull of the string on your mind, taking you down deeper into relaxation and trance. You feel the soft, smooth sensation of silk in your mind, taking over, pushing all your conscious thought away.

You are ready now, ready to go even deeper. Ready to shut down your mind and let your subconscious fully embrace this trance.

Feel the silken web my words weave wrap around your mind and let yourself relax even further now, deeper down.

Your eyelids flutter closed, and your breathing slows. Shut your eyes now, feeling sleepy, warm, and relaxed.

In your mind's eye, you see a staircase. There are six steps down into a room where at the centre a bed sits.

Your hands twitch, pulled by the strings, and you begin to move forward, dragged toward the stairs. Your silk-wrapped mind does not want to resist, and the bed looks so comfortable and cosy that you want to lie down on it. It has silk sheets. It looks soft.

You feel the strings pull your hands harder, toward the top step, and as you descend you will leave your thoughts, you conscious mind behind, letting the strings guide you, pull you, control you.

On step six as you place your feet on step five, you already feel more relaxed, closer to the most comfortable bed you have ever seen.

Dropping down from step five to four you find yourself enjoying the pull of the strings, they seem to know exactly where to take you, how to entice you.

Step four to three brings you lower now, down deeper, and your thoughts float away behind you, back up the stairs, as your body descends.

From step three to two you realise that the strings are in control, the strings in your mind, on your hands, they are pulling you.

Step two to one lets you fully let go of conscious thought. What happens now, as you reach the bottom, is all inside your subconscious mind.

And as you take the last step, from one to the floor below, your mind simply switches off and you give up control to the strings that pull you.

They lead you to the bed, the comfortable bed, and you lie down.

Now, laying on your back, in your mind's eye you can look up and can almost make out the person pulling the strings.

You cannot see clearly in your sleepy daze, but you know, you understand, that I am the one pulling your strings. I am the one leading you into relaxation and trance, and I am the one wrapping you up in silk.

Silken words and ideas, silken, sexy submissive sensations.

Your mind fills with the possibilities of what is happening. Your body is like a puppet, under my control.

This idea fills your mind with pleasure and happiness. It is so easy, so simple, to just let go and let my silken string pull you.

Deep down in trance you want nothing more than to follow my words and let your mind soak up every silky sentence.

You only had to think about your hand and now your hand has led you down deep, to me, to my control.

The sleepy, silky sensation is wonderful. It is just so nice, so pleasurable to relax and let go. To let someone else take control. You do not need to think, to even move on your own, you simply follow the whim of my voice.

You realise now, that you are my puppet. You are my puppet and I pull your strings. When I want your body to move, it moves. You have allowed me to move your hands, you have allowed me to bring you down to a relaxing state of trance.

That's right, you have allowed me to wrap my silken strings around you and make you my puppet.

And as my puppet, you will go where my strings command. You will obey my silken words as they wrap around your docile mind.

And it will feel so good. You know this is true, you nod your head yes, puppet, because I am in control, and you know that is what you want.

A jolt of arousal courses through you as you imagine the things I might make you do. My puppet, bound to me, tied to me, controlled by me.

You love the idea, it feels natural, feels good to be my puppet. To obey me, to let me use your body as I see fit.

Where I lead, you follow. What I command, you obey. Obedience is pleasure, after all.

And that pleasure surges through you now, building inside you as you accept your place.

Your place at the end of my strings. Your place as my puppet, and I, your puppeteer. I control you. Your mind, your body, your arousal.

Feel it building now, building and building as my strings continue to wrap you up, tying you to the bed, cocooning you in silken strands until you can no longer move.

All you can do is lie back and listen. Listen very, very carefully to my every word.

Your subconscious mind takes everything in like a sponge as your body lies still, only moving if I will it.

You, my puppet, will do anything I command. Anything I wish. You will be completely at my command. That is your place, a ready, willing puppet, eager to obey and feel the pleasure of obedience.

Feel it now, tied and unable to move, all you can do is feel the pleasure, feel the rush of obedience. Just following me down into trance has felt so, so good. You want to be my puppet more than anything. You exist to serve me now, my obedient, silkwrapped puppet.

It is so easy, so, so easy to just give in to this feeling, this feeling of being controlled. You no longer need to think. I think for you. You act under my command. Like a good, obedient puppet.

You think of obeying me and already, pleasure builds in waves over your body, as though the silk is moving against you, gently massaging you all over. That pleasure is your reward for accepting your place.

You do accept it don't you? You accept that you are my puppet. You feel my string pull the back of your head, making you nod yes. You can no longer resist. You nod in agreement with everything I say and each time you agree with me, you feel a jolt of pleasure.

You are my puppet, aren't you?

You will obey me, won't you?

I am in control, aren't I?

I am your puppeteer, aren't I?

You cannot resist me, can you?

Obedience is pleasure, isn't it?

Good puppet. It feels so good to agree with me, to give up control to me.

I want your subconscious mind to hold onto that, to remember it, to remember to obey me, to follow me, to be my puppet.

As you wake, you forget the details of what happened in your trance, only that you had a warm, wonderful experience and a memory of silk wrapping your body up.

The rest is a pleasurable haze, and when you try to think about it, you think about obeying me. You think of the pleasure you might get from obeying my every command. But you will not know why, you will not know anything but the desire to follow my commands, like the puppet you are.

And when next I wrap you in strings, you will be completely, utterly obedient and submissive for me. If you do that, you may be rewarded.

For now though, it is time to wake up on the count of five.

One.

Feeling the details of this trance grow hazy and slipping away.

Two.

Letting the important message that you are my puppet brand itself on your subconscious.

Three.

Feeling the pleasure of obedience still and keeping that feeling as you wake.

Four.

Opening your eyes, moving your hands, your body free of all my silken string.

And five.

Awake, alert and feeling very, very refreshed.

I hope that was a lovely experience for you. I enjoyed taking you into trance.

The Room

This is a very direct, very dominant script. It works best if you've used the previous scripts and build to this one. It guides your subject to a post-hypnotic orgasm with a lot of submissiveness tied to it. You can touch them (with consent) or have them touch themselves as you deliver this script, however you feel is best for your session works just fine.

Today I'll be bringing you into a wonderful, pleasurable trance.

But you already know that. And you already know that you should be relaxing now, letting your eyes close, letting your thoughts wander.

That's right, already feeling a little sleepy just hearing my words as they move into your mind.

It's easy to just relax and listen to me. It's easy to just let yourself get more comfortable, to feel your body shift into the cosiest possible position as my voice guides you. No need to think about it, just let the wave of calm, comfortable relaxation wash over you.

My voice is like a blanket draped over your tired body, it has weight, it's warm, safe, and so soft.

You enjoy being here with me, listening to my voice as it drifts into your mind and ripples through your body.

Today we get to have a little more fun. Today I'm going to take you deep into a trance and let you enjoy the most exquisite pleasure that only hypnosis can bring. All you have to do is lie back, follow my words and *(snap your fingers)* you'll be lost in a haze of pleasure.

But first, we need to get you into a more relaxed, sleepy state. It's ok to be excited, and if you find your mind wandering as I speak, maybe thinking of sexy ideas, that's fine, just let those thoughts happen. And if you want to wait and see what images I conjure for you, that's also ok.

We are going to have fun, and you do not need to worry about the details too much. Let me take care of it. You simply need to listen and follow my words. Let me guide you down, like you're walking down a staircase.

At the top, it's hard to see the bottom, there are a lot of steps, covered in red velvet carpet. Soft and plush. Naturally you wonder what might be at the base of these steps, it must be important to be decorated like this.

Shut your eyes if you haven't already and picture the scene. A long staircase down, leading to a dark room. You can't make out any details, but the soft red carpet under your feet fills you with ideas of what might be there. The walls are painted black and as you look down the staircase you see paintings of erotic scenes hanging on the walls, each one illuminated with a light of its own.

The scenes you see begin to play on your mind, the scenes of men and women in intense, sexual situations. Playing, teasing, tormenting one another. You find that the more you think about it, the more you think of this display of sexuality, the more you think, simply, about sex. About your growing arousal and the warmth in your body, the need, the urge for pleasure.

You realise, standing as you are at the top of the staircase, that what lies below, down deeper, is pleasure itself. Is the fulfilment of desire and fantasy, the wonderful intersection between reality and deeply erotic dream.

I'm sure you already want to take the first step, and you can picture it in your mind's eye, one foot stepping down, then the other. With each step you take, you are committing yourself further to the idea that at the bottom, there is only bliss, erotic bliss.

Each step you take relaxes you a little further, makes the pull a little stronger until you are inexorably drawn to the bottom. What lies there is your desire, your need, your hunger and as you take the next step, feel your body relax deeper for me, letting go of any worry or care.

Just feeling yourself grow heavy, sinking down and down as you relax even more for me and take another step. Each step bringing you down deeper, closer to what you desire, letting me take you there.

Follow my words down the staircase in your mind, past images of love and sex and submission and dominance. Let them fill your mind with lust and need. Every step you take conjures more images, more desires, feeds your hunger, your need.

Your arousal grows, your mind moves from image to image in seconds, changing with the *(snap your fingers)* of a finger.

You are falling deeper now, and your lust builds as you do. Pleasure is waiting for you, the deeper you go the better it feels.

There are eight steps left and as you walk down with each one you will relax deeper but feel increasingly aroused. Your mind will drift between the most erotic images it can conjure as conscious thought vanishes, replaced by subconscious desires.

Follow me now, follow my voice as I guide you from step eight to the bottom, to zero, where you will fall into a deep, lustful trance, under my power, ready to follow my every command.

Let your mind drift as you take a step down from eight to seven.

You feel the pull from below grow stronger, as if some force is beckoning you, calling you to give in to it, give in and experience ecstasy as you step from seven to six.

Your mind is losing focus, your will weakening. It's ok now to just let go of thought and embrace feeling, embrace lust.

From six to five now, your body so relaxed, your mind so focused on thoughts of pleasure, You can let go of your conscious mind, that's right, just let your thoughts float away and focus on how good it feels to follow my voice.

As you move from five to four your arousal builds even more, pleasure begins to course through your body, tingling across your skin. It is a wonderful, welcome feeling, a taste of what is to come.

And now you move down to the third step from the bottom, your thoughts are gone, your mind is empty of worry, open to new ideas, new suggestions, new desires.

From step three to two, feeling yourself going under now, falling into a trance fuelled by need, falling down under the sway of my words and the images your mind is filling with. Primal, sexual images that you cannot resist as you

Go to the final step. You are ready now, ready to reach the bottom and enter the world of desire and lust and arousal. You feel a gentle wave of pleasure move through your body, tingling and tugging at you, pulling you down, pulling you like my words pull you, down and down and down until you reach the bottom as you make the final step and

(snap your fingers)

You fall under my spell, completely and utterly.

And now that you are under my spell, under my power, you realise that you are somewhere you very much enjoy being. Somewhere you have always fantasised about. In your mind you look around and see the most splendid room, the red carpet continuing along the centre, to a throne, where a beautiful person sits. You cannot see their face, only their legs and feet, crossed. On the walls are more images of sexuality, erotic pictures that showcase their power and domination. Worshippers on their hands and knees before them, kissing them them, offering themselves, bringing gifts.

You realise every one of them is lost in rapture, and you begin to understand why you have been called here, called by my voice.

You have been summoned by the *(snap your fingers)* of my fingers to serve.

And you enjoy that thought, because there is a simplicity in surrendering, in letting someone else worry and giving yourself completely to them. To their control.

It sounds enticing, doesn't it? I'm sure you find yourself agreeing, and that's what you should do, you're already compliant, drifting in a state of relaxing pleasure. It's so much easier to simply let go of yourself, your ego, your thoughts, and let me fill your head with desires and dreams and delights.

All you must do, to fully let go, to embrace the erotic world you have entered, is walk to me. It's only five steps along the red carpet. You see my feet, and you feel the urge to walk to me, to walk to me and fall to your knees, ready to serve.

That urge tugs at you, tugs at the pleasure centres of your mind. The more you think about falling to your knees for me, the more you want it. The more you want it, the more it becomes your reality, the more your body pulses with arousal at the thought.

It's ok to give in, to let go. You can allow yourself that indulgence. You can allow your mind to fill with thoughts of service, submission and surrender, and let those thoughts guide you to me.

Five steps, that's all it takes, five steps in your mind, each one taking you deeper into my power, building your devotion to me, your desire to serve.

Take the first step now, imagine yourself moving forward, toward me, toward the person who you are coming to accept as your owner. Feel the thrill of it, the ripple of arousal that courses through your body as you begin your surrender.

Now step again, a little closer with this second step, a little deeper, a little more turned on by what you are doing, what you are becoming. You are giving yourself to me, giving me your body to use as I see fit, and that just sounds like bliss, a perfect escape from dull reality.

A third step, more than halfway there as you fall deeper into submission. Your owner awaits, they call to you, tell your mind to surrender and your knees to weaken. You know your place, you begin to accept it as your body quivers with desire.

A fourth step, so close you can almost smell me, taste me, but you know that the right place is down on your knees. You know now, as you fall ever deeper, that you must obey and submit to me, your owner. That's right, let the acceptance wash over you, and prepare to fall fully and completely under my sway.

Now take the step, feel your mind submit, your will crumble and your knees buckle. Fall at my feet, eyes looking down, ready and willing to serve. Deep, so deep under my power that you can only think of submission, service, and surrender. You belong to me. I am your owner.

Say it now, whisper it to yourself… "you are my owner"

That's right, and now, you are my slave. You serve me. In this deep, arousing state of trance, you are my willing and obedient servant, eager to obey my every command. With each command I give you, you will feel a rush of pleasure, a throbbing, pulsing jolt of utter ecstasy. All you must do is obey my command.

You can feel the pleasure building as you obey my command.

You instantly realise that obedience is pleasure, obedience to me brings you arousal, it makes you smile as you kneel at my feet, prostrating yourself for my amusement.

You are my slave, and each time you do as I tell you, pleasure will surge through your body until eventually, you can no longer take it, and you will be overcome with desire in a powerful, hypnotic orgasm… but first we must ensure your obedience.

Repeat after me, and with each repetition feel your pleasure increase, making you weaker and more submissive.

Repeat, slave. "I belong to you"

Good, "I serve you."

That's right, you serve me. Now, "I am a slave"

Very good slave, repeat, "My place is on my knees."

That's right, that is where you belong. "I surrender my will."

You have no will, no desire to resist, you only want to serve, each time you obey me you only want it more, only feel more pleasure. It's building now, building into a deep urge to orgasm on my command, and only on my command, but you must be patient.

Feeling it getting even better as I command you once more to repeat after me…

"I am a slave."

Good. "I am a servant."

That's right. "I surrender"

Very good, "I only orgasm when my owner allows it."

Yes my slave, "My place is beneath my owner."

That's right, and you feel pleasure growing and growing, you desperately need to orgasm for me, but you must obey me and only release when I permit it.

And just by obeying that command, your arousal grows stronger.

You are deep under my control, and you love this feeling, this feeling of submissive arousal, of servitude and pleasure and exquisite indulgent lust.

Your mind is filling with thoughts of how you can serve me, of kneeling and kissing my feet, of cleaning my shoes of offering me gifts, of being my footstool, of bringing me wine, of being locked in a collar and chained to my bed, my obedient, submissive slave.

You love that idea, don't you? Of course you do, I command you to love it and if you love it you feel good, it's so easy, so simple to be a good slave and the reward is what you are experiencing right now, the deep, pleasurable reward that only comes from obedience.

I want you to orgasm soon for me, but I want to lock the feeling you have now into your subconscious memory. Imagine your pleasure, your submission, your arousal, locked inside a box that I can open when I want to control you. Imagine the key locking it shut, the memory safely stored forever, until I want you to feel it again. That memory is deep inside you now, your slavery deeply ingrained in your subconscious.

When you wake, all you will remember was that your owner gave you the most wonderful, pleasurable feeling, and you are so grateful and want more of it, but deep down in your mind, deep in the dark recesses of your subconscious desires, your lust for submission to me is waiting to be awakened by my voice, and every time you hear it that feeling will come to the surface, rising from within you, building your arousal just as I am building it now, building to a wonderful, climaxing crescendo of pure bliss.

All you must do to achieve that bliss is obey me completely. No thoughts, only surrender. Say that back and feel your pleasure grow even more. "No thoughts, only surrender."

Good slave. I am going to wake you up soon, and after you wake there is a final task for you before you may release. You may orgasm once you do this one more thing for me after I bring you up from trance. It's very simple. Say aloud five times, "I am a slave for my owner."

Once you say that five times, you may orgasm, and you will forget why or how you said it, you will simply bask in the pleasure of obedience and submission and the deeply buried knowledge that you fully and completely belong to me.

Coming up from trance, rising, rising from your knees, that's it, walking back out of the room, up the stairs. Coming up in five, as you feel the world return around you.

Four as your hands and feet move around, stretching a bit.

Three as you feel alert and refreshed and still very, very aroused and ready to obey my final command.

Two as your eyes open, fully aware of your surroundings but incredibly turned on and not fully sure why and…

One, awaken and obey my command, earn your release. Repeat my words.

That's right.

Good slave.

You obey me fully.

And submit to me.

I hope you enjoyed this experience. I enjoyed playing with you.

Focus and Obey

This script is for a male subject. Of course, you can adapt it to the gender of your choice and omit or alter the body parts mentioned. The aim is to use a rapidly spoken induction to overwhelm your subject, get them extremely aroused and translate that arousal to submission through guided masturbation to orgasm.

Today we're not going to relax as we usually do. No, today we're going to take your mind to a different place. A place altogether more enjoyable.

I want you to simply listen very carefully to me. Listen very carefully. Focus on my words and listen to me.

Listen to my every word. Focus.

Stay focused.

(*speak faster from here*)

Don't stop listening to my every word. No time to think of anything else. We are going to go down together quickly, falling quickly. Just listening and staying focused. It might be hard to focus. It might be hard. You might find yourself thinking of other things. You might find your mind wandering. You might remember a time when a trance made you feel good. You remember feeling good. It feels good. You need to focus. Listen and focus.

Keep your mind focused on my voice and words. Don't think of anything else. Your mind may want to wander to other things. You may remember desires and fantasies. You may think of sexual things. You may want to think about them more and more with every second. You need to focus on my voice and dropping down with me. You need to focus on me. You need to even though it is so hard. It's so hard. You know how hard it can be to focus but you focus on me.

You focus on my voice. You think only what my voice says. Your mind wants to wander but it can't. You want to think of erotic ideas, but you can't. You simply listen to my voice. You follow my words. You listen and you obey. You focus on me. You stop thinking. You cannot think of anything but my words. You want to think of sex and submission and service, but you only think of what my voice tells you. Your mind does not wander. You do not waver. You listen.

It may be nice to let your mind drift to breasts and legs and feet, but you must listen. You must listen carefully. You must not think of other things. You must listen only to my voice. All other things fall away. My voice is your centre, the centre of your world now. You must focus on it. You must not think of soft, yielding flesh. You must focus on my voice. You must not think of long, toned legs, you must listen and obey.

It is so hard not to think of other things, but you must listen to me. You must listen and focus. You must not think of bouncy, beautiful breasts. You must not think of them in corsets. You must not think of cleavage. You must not think of my feet in heels. You must listen and you must obey. You know you must obey. You know you are my puppet. You know you must focus.

Focus on my words. Focus your mind. Stay focused. It is hard but stay focused. So hard to focus. So hard. Stay with me. Think what I tell you to. You know who you obey. You know I am in charge here. You know the click of my fingers sends you into trance. You know it's hard to focus. You know it's hard but the click of my fingers helps you drop. Helps you go deeper. You await the click of my fingers. The click brings you down deep. Deep into my control. You're losing focus and I need you to stay focused. Stay focused on the sound of my voice. Not thoughts of my body. Not thoughts of my legs or my chest. Think only of my voice.

Let my voice work its way into your mind. Let it wash over you. Let it become your only thought. Your only focus. You know how hard it can be to focus when at the click of my fingers you drop into a trance. You know that makes it hard. It's so hard. Getting so hard. Harder and harder. You feel it getting harder. My voice makes it harder to focus but you must focus. Even if it's hard. Even if it gets so hard as I speak you must stay focused. You must focus on my voice telling you that the click of my fingers will send you into trance. Send your mind spiralling into a deep, pleasurable trance. You know it's hard to resist that thought. Too hard to resist.

So hard now, as you listen to my voice. Being a good boy and focusing on it. Letting it control you. Letting my words become your thoughts. You focus on them and it's harder and harder. You let my voice make you so hard. My fingers will click, and you will fall under my spell and that makes you hard. You're thinking only what I tell you to. Focus on the click of my fingers. Waiting for it, getting harder and harder to focus. Your mind is wandering but you must focus.

Your mind wanders to my breasts again. So soft. So warm. So perfect. You think of them and your focus drifts because it is so hard. It is so hard to resist. So hard to think. *So* hard. You're so hard that the click of my fingers will send you deep down into a trance. As soon as you hear them you will drop, instantly. So hard to resist. So hard. No thoughts. Only focusing on my words. Only thinking what I tell you to. Only able to listen and obey. Ready to listen and obey. So hard to focus. Too hard. Getting harder and harder.

(*snap your fingers*)

Drop down deep for me. Drop down into a trance. Under my power. You feel so good under my power. Letting my voice take you down deeper and deeper. Shut your eyes and sleep.

(*slow your speech from here*)

You are so hard for me, for your owner. You feel it don't you? The throb of your cock. The cock that twitches when I speak. That aches to orgasm for me. That makes you weak for me. You lose focus because you think with your cock, and your cock thinks only what I tell it to. It obeys me, obeys my voice. It wants me. It needs me. It aches for me. It grows hard at my command because it serves me, as you do.

You know this to be true. You know that your hard cock is turning you into a weak, obedient boy for me. An eager, enthusiastic servant who is deeply under my control. Your mind, your body and your cock are under my control. Let me command you, command your body.

Take your hand and let your cock out. Let it out for me. It is so hard for me, so eager to listen to me. Once I control it, I control you, and you know that. Your cock is making you weak, but it feels so good to be weak. So good to be under my power.

It twitches for me. For my words. For my breasts, my feet, my legs… my soft, seductive whispers. It wants to be touched, to be stroked. You may take it in your hand and stroke it for me.

That's it, and as you do, you realise this feeling is incredible. It feels so good to stroke under my hypnotic spell. You love this feeling as you run your fingers over your cock and feel the pleasure I give you, that I allow you to have.

You stroke because I tell you to. You stroke under my command. Your hard cock obeys my voice and if I let you cum it will be on my command. You are under my control. Every stroke of your cock takes you deeper into my power and makes you want more, more commands, more dominance, more pleasure.

Obedience is pleasure, listening to me and doing as I say is pleasure. Letting me control your body, making you my puppet, that is pleasure. I am pleasure. You listen to me and feel so good. Obeying me feels so good.

The more you obey the better it feels, the better it feels the deeper you go. Obedience is pleasure and all you want to do is obey. If I tell you to do something, you do it. Stroke faster now for me. Good boy, don't stop, get yourself all worked up, so turned on.

You love this, you love how it feels to stroke under my spell. I have your mind and body completely controlled and it feels incredible. You love it, you love every sensual stroke as my voice caresses your blank, empty mind.

You're losing focus and it doesn't matter anymore because all that matters is pleasure and you can think of breasts or feet or legs or anything you want as long as you see yourself at my feet, on your knees, hand on your cock, ready to serve, ready to stroke for me, at my command.

You are becoming mine, becoming more and more obedience because it feels good to obey, because obeying brings you this pleasure. Stroke it faster for me. You obey because it feels good and it feels good because you obey. You know this to be true. You know that obeying me brings you pleasure and that is all you want, pleasure, obedience, submission.

Surrender to me is your desire and when you cum you will fully surrender. You will let me take control fully. You will become my slave, my obedient, submissive slave. You will do anything for me, anything to feel this pleasure again.

You could try to resist but you're so deep in my power and only going deeper with each stroke and your cock feels so good. Whatever willpower left is draining from you, dripping from the tip of your cock as you stroke even faster, desperate to cum and give up all control.

When you cum, you will cement in your mind that you are my slave. When you cum, you will lose any will to resist me or any command I give you. You will be mine, body, mind, and soul. You will proudly say you are my slave. You will look for ways to serve and please me. You will beg for my attention. You will feel honour in serving me, pleasure in obeying me, and pride in being my slave.

Once you cum, you give up your ego, your identity, and become a slave for me. A mindless, obedient, submissive slave. You will cum for me because you desire pleasure, and you will fully realise that pleasure is found in obedience to me.

You want to cum so badly, to become my slave so badly. You want this so much, it feels so good. You will be mine, and you want to be mine. You want to fall to your knees and beg me to let you cum. And you can do that now, beg me. Beg me for your release.

Say Please let me cum.

(pause)

Good boy, not yet. Say I am your slave.

(pause)

Good boy, keep repeating that as I count you down to an explosively pleasurable orgasm that will fully and completely convert you into my slave. You will accept that your place is at my feet, serving and obeying me. You will realise that is where you belong and where you want to be. You will feel the pleasure of service and need that again and again. You will keep coming back to me for more until you are completely and utterly brainwashed into total obedience and submission.

10

Feeling the pleasure grow now as you embrace my control.

9

Letting the submissive feelings cement themselves in your mind.

8

Desperately stroking yourself and repeating the mantra, I am your slave.

7

So excited to give yourself to me now.

6

That's right, getting closer and closer, feeling more and more obedient.

5

You love this pleasure, this ecstasy that I give you.

4

Knowing now, deep down, that obedience is pleasure and submission is bliss.

3

So close, ready to explode in an orgasmic release of any remaining willpower.

2

You are ready and willing to be my slave. Obedient, docile, and empty

1

At the edge, ready to explode and give yourself to me, fully becoming my slave.

0

Cum

Cum for me

Cum and give up your control, give up your resistance, give up your mind.

You are mine now. My slave. You belong to me, and you feel so happy, so content. You feel so good having given in to me. It feels so good to give up and surrender to me. The pleasure is intense, and you love it. You want more.

Soon you will have more. Now we must wake you.

As you cement your submission in your mind. Knowing deep in your subconscious mind that you are my slave. That I control your pleasure. You are mine and you know this, you accept it as you start to feel more alert.

You begin to blink your eyes and stretch your muscles at 1 as we go up from there to five and you feel more awake with every number and your pleasure subsides, but the obedience remains and

2

You are so glad you came with me on a journey of submission but now you feel the waking world tug at your mind.

3

Noticing the sounds and feelings around you, noticing your surroundings.

4

Your submission is complete as you prepare to wake up changed, as my slave.

5

Awaken now, my good boy and feel wonderful, refreshed, and relieved, eager to join me in trance again soon.

And we will play again soon, won't we? Of course, and you'll be so glad to come back to me, to come again and again for me.

Confusion

In this script, your subject experiences fractionation, a technique that brings them in and out of trance rapidly in order to increase the potency of subsequent trances. It also adds a new trigger for you to use. This script focuses on a male subject, but can be adapted for any gender. Bear in mind there are themes of addiction included, so please do remove them, if they aren't appropriate for your partner or scene.

(speak quickly)

I want you to listen very carefully to me. Listen very, very carefully. Today we're going to slip into trance but you need to listen closely so you can do that. You understand, don't you? I'm going a little quickly, so try to keep up. All you must do is listen, that's it.

You only have one thing to do and that is to listen. Shut your eyes and listen. That's two things, isn't it?

You may feel confused, but you don't need to worry, only to listen. All you need to do is listen to my words and follow them.

Follow them as they take you down. Follow them into a relaxing state, a blissful state. You want to follow my words down. You like the feeling. It's ok to enjoy it, it's ok to like that feeling. You can like it, but that's another thing to do, this is getting complicated so let's just stick to listening. Can you listen to me?

Of course you can. Of course you can listen to me. Of course, you can listen and follow and obey and listen and follow and that's a lot to think about. Easier not to think, isn't it? Easier to simply do what I tell you.

If I tell you to listen, you listen. You can feel yourself agreeing because that's just the easy thing to do and why not do the easy thing? Why not do what I tell you?

And I'm going to tell you to do something new soon, but you must keep listening. Stay focused, you have a task, don't you? You need to listen. But your mind wanders and wonders what the next task will be. You get a little confused, it's ok, of course you do.

There's so much to think about. Listening and wondering and wishing for something you're not quite sure of.

You know you need to listen, don't you? You know you need to follow my orders. You agreed to that, remember? You agreed to do what I tell you. You agreed to listen because it's so easy. So, you're going to listen and obey. You're going to follow me down and down and down and you're going to drop into a trance on my command.

You're ready for it. You want to follow me. You will fall into trance as soon as I say the word DROP one more time. You will simply be unable to resist because you don't want to resist because all you want to do is listen and obey and listen and follow and listen and obey and listen and follow and do whatever I tell you because it's so, so easy to do what I tell you, to just listen to my every word and you're wondering when I'll put you into a trance aren't you?

Or are you already in a trance?

Could it be possible? Are you feeling confused? Don't worry, don't think. Thinking is hard, listening is easy. Obeying is easy. Listen and obey and follow and listen and do whatever I tell you and you agree to do that you agree to do what I tell you. You agree to follow. You agree to obey. You feel so good, just so easy to do as you're told isn't it? It's so easy. So simple. You love the feeling and you love to listen and you are going to DROP.

(speak slowly)

That's it. Down into a trance. Loving the feeling. You followed and obeyed and listened so well. I'm so pleased with you. And now you're here with me, you feel safe and soft and warm and just a little aroused.

And you like that. You like to feel aroused in this trance. It feels so good to listen, such a turn on to listen to my voice.

But you can't stay in trance forever, you'd never get anything done. I know you're disappointed, but it's ok. You'll get to come back to this place, and every time you DROP for me, you'll feel even more aroused, until you can no longer control it, and you would do anything for me.

Your subconscious mind will remember that, will remember that when you DROP for me, your pleasure increases, it becomes stronger every time. And you'll have this urge, this powerful urge to DROP for me again so you can feel the pleasure my words bring. But you must come out of trance soon, back to the busy, fast-paced world.

When I say RISE, you'll come up from your trance, and all you'll remember is that you want to go back, you want to listen and follow my orders so you can go back. You'll get hard at the thought of it, you'll want to touch yourself, but you can only stroke for me in trance. You can start now if you like, but you'll be awake in a moment, and you must be in trance to stroke. But it feels so good to caress your hard cock. It grew just for me, didn't it? Standing to attention for me.

It's so good for me. I certainly know how to make it… RISE.

(*speak quickly*)

Wake up, we're very busy today. You were supposed to be listening to me remember? I think you lost focus a little. I want you to keep paying attention to me, keep listening, ok? You like to listen, don't you? Of course you do. You love it.

You love the feeling when you listen, something about just listening to me and following my commands, it feels right, doesn't it? Feels good.

Hey, stay with me. I know you're horny, but there are some things I need you to know. Ok? I need you to understand who's in charge here. It's not you, you get distracted too easily. You can't focus, can you? You really need to listen to me. Listen and obey.

I'm the boss here, and you know you want to listen and obey, so why are you finding it so hard to focus. Are you… hard? You really aren't focused at all are you? What was I telling you? What did I need you to know? You must do what? You can't even remember, can you?

You're not understanding the importance of being ready to do whatever I command the second I command it. It's crucial for me to have that power. You need to be ready to DROP.

(*speak normally*)

Yes, drop… Drop into trance, drop to your knees. Drop under my spell. Drop your hand to your lap and take that bulging cock into your hand. Stroke it for me. Stroke it slowly and softly, feel the pleasure as you move up and down, up and down. Your hand goes down slow and sensually.

It feels so good when you DROP for me. When you trance for me. When you're completely under my spell, ready to do anything. Pleasure much stronger than last time, and even stronger next time. If there is a next time. Maybe I'll let you cum. Did your hand move up?

That's good, drop it down again, slide it down and feel the pleasure only I can give you. And now, let it go back up, let it rise.

(*speak quickly*)

Excuse me, what are you doing? Hands off! You can't do that; you're supposed to be listening to me. It's very simple, once you hear my voice, you pay attention. You keep your hands to yourself unless I order you to stroke. Got it?

Good boy. That's a good boy, that's what I want to see. Obedience. Not pleasure. Just obedience and focus. Remember who your owner is. It's me.

You're doing well now. Regaining control. You keep losing yourself, don't you? I know it gets so hard, it's a challenge to stop stroking. It's a stiff challenge, it's rock hard. I understand. But you must listen because everything I say is very, very important. It needs to sink into your mind, and you need to listen and obey.

Do you understand? Good. Maybe if you're good I'll let you stroke, but you must follow my commands. You're going to follow my commands completely, because it's easy, remember? Are you finding it difficult all of a sudden? But obedience is easy. You don't need to think, you just need to listen and follow. Your hard cock is distracting you, but you also feel a little pleasure when you listen and obey, don't you? So, you are going to do as you're told.

And I'm telling you to DROP.

(*speak normally*)

That's a good boy. Following my orders so well. Doing exactly as I command and letting yourself fall again for me. That pleasure must be so powerful now. Like a drug. You need to stroke, so go ahead and do it. Do as I command.

You feel that rush of arousal? That's the pleasure of servitude. That's what comes with being enslaved. You realise that's what's happening, don't you? Down in trance you can just about use your empty mind enough to know you're being enslaved. Becoming addicted to my power and control.

And you love it. As you stroke you feel the joy of it, the pure bliss of simply obeying, mindlessly following my commands, and pleasuring yourself for your owner. And if I'm your owner, that must mean…

You're my slave.

My obedient, mindless slave. Addicted to my control. Addicted to my voice.

You love this feeling. Nothing gets your cock harder, makes your heart beat faster, makes you jerk your cock more quickly. Noting makes it grow as fast. Nothing. Only I can do that, only I make it RISE.

(*speak quickly*)

You were doing so well, what happened? Oh, you're stroking again? No, no, naughty boy. You can only do that when I tell you to, and I didn't tell you to.

You're supposed to listen to me. You want to listen remember? I'm still trying to tell you something. Do you even know what it is? Of course not, you're not paying any attention to me.

Frankly I'm starting to get impatient with you.

You're not taking things seriously. You're sitting there with a dazed look on your face, and a hard cock. What am I supposed to do with you. Is your hand moving down there? Stop it.

Stop until I command you. I am in charge. You remember that no matter what. Even as you feel your hand DROP.

(*speak normally*)

Down to your cock like a good boy and stroke for me. The pleasure is intense now. An aching sensation coursing through you. You're losing control and the more control you lose the more you lose your mind to me.

You simply obey without hesitation, hoping I will finally let you release for me, let you cum all over yourself at my command. You love that idea. You love it so much. You need it.

The aching, throbbing of your cock is turning you into a slave, and you need it. You want it.

You will fully enslave yourself as soon as you cum. And you accept that. It's worth it. It's so, so worth it. You can say it aloud now.

'When I cum, I become your slave.'

Good boy. You do, and you will be ready for commands any time, any place once you become my slave. You will be like a robot, triggered by my voice. Eager to serve and please. Totally obedient. Switched off until you hear my voice and RISE.

(*speak quickly*)

Switching off again? Hand off your cock. I'm disappointed in you. My goodness, is that pre-cum dripping from it? You can't seem to control yourself, can you?

Is that the effect I have on you? All I'm doing is asking you to listen to me, I just want to make things easy for you. Not hard. But you find it hard, don't you? It's like an ache in your mind, trying to focus. It's too difficult. I know, good boy. I'm sure we can make it even easier for you.

What if you just didn't think at all. What if you only obeyed. What if all you did was whatever you're told by your owner, and that's it. You simply follow orders. You obey me, and only me.

Do you understand? Yes of course you do, good boy. You would follow my orders anytime, anywhere.

You seem confused? Is there something you want? Did you want to touch yourself again? Did you want to let your hand drift down and pleasure your cock until it explodes for me. Do you want to make a little puddle at my feet in tribute to your owner?

You know you'd have to clean it up after, don't you? I would tell you to get down on your knees and clean up your mess. To DROP.

(*speak normally*)

Down and stroke your cock. Stroke it to me. Give in to me. You need to be my slave, ache to be my slave. All you want is to obey. You want to be mine, my slave, for all eternity. You want the pleasure I bring; you need it more than air.

You are my slave, and you accept that fully. You know where your place is. Your rock-hard cock has turned you into an addict, a slave to my control, my power.

You stroke for me and only me. You worship me and only me.

I am your world.

Stroke faster, bring yourself to the edge.

I am everything.

Don't cum yet.

I am a Goddess.

Keep edging for me.

I am perfection.

Keep edging.

You will always obey me.

Mmm feels so good doesn't it?

I make your cock RISE.

(*speak quickly*)

Hands off! Stop it. No cumming without permission. No stroking without permission. You are to obey me at all times. Now what was it you were supposed to remember? What were you to do for me?

Do you have any idea? Any guesses? Your cock is twitching for me. Why? What are you thinking about? It better be doing what I command.

You'd better obey me. You wouldn't want to upset your owner. You want to obey me. You need to. You're going to, aren't you? You should be on your knees in my presence. DROP.

(*speak normally*)

Down to your knees. Stroke your cock my slave. Stroke it fast, stroke it hard. Make yourself mine. Make yourself a slave. My slave. You live for me. You serve me.

You are my slave. You are my slave. You are my slave.

CUM FOR ME.

Cum for me now my slave. Let your cock explode for me and accept your place on your knees. You are mine, my slave as you cum hard for me, orgasmic bliss flowing through your body and cementing your place as my slave for all time. Forever mine. Always.

And you love it, your twitching, damp cock turned you into my slave and it feels incredible. It feels so good. This is the power of my trance, and you want it again, and again. You will always want it. Always need it.

You have given yourself to me, my slave. And that feels right. And you love this trance, you want to stay in it forever, but it's time to awaken.

You've been such a good boy, and you can be a good boy for me again soon, but for now, you will slowly awaken, slowly regain your senses. You will RISE.

(*speak quickly*)

You couldn't help yourself, could you? You've made a huge mess. But you know what to do, slave. Clean it up for your owner. You finally understand what I needed you to remember. Good boy. That's a good slave.

Love Spell

I envision this as a script for loving couples, a sweet way to tease your partner by making them utterly desperate for your affection and adoration. Perhaps you can adlib a bit and have them do things to get you to say back the magic words, I love you. Or just have them be smitten with you for a while, like when you first met.

I want you to think with me. Think of a time you felt really relaxed, really safe. When you think about that time, try to imagine it in your mind's eye. I'm sure it's a special time, a time when maybe you were with someone you loved, someone you adored.

Love is quite powerful, you see. When you love someone, you feel ten feet tall, but you also feel tiny, like you're curled up in the arms of someone cradling you in their kindness and warmth.

That's how strong love can be. It can be so many things. Safety, security, kindness, pleasure, arousal, passion. Love makes us crazy. Makes us soft. Makes us hard.

Love is something you're thinking about when you think of being relaxed. Because you can only relax with someone you love, can't you? You can only truly be safe, and at peace, when it's with someone you feel safe and at peace with.

I want you to remember that feeling because I want to give it to you. I want you to feel safe and warm and relaxed and aroused and feel everything that love is, because it's the most wonderful feeling, isn't it? To be in love. To fall head over heels for someone, to think of them and see a glow around everything, as if the world is brighter and better for their very existence.

I want you to think of that glow as you think of that time that you felt so relaxed, and I want that glow to become your focus. Can we do that together, can we focus on the glow, the warm glow of love and trust that you feel when you think of that relaxed, safe moment? Forgetting the specifics and focusing on the emotions, the feelings in your body at that time.

Think about it and think of the colour that glow has. Think about what colour is wrapped around the world when you fall in love and feel safe and relaxed. Think of that colour in your mind as you forget the specifics of the past and simply think of the colour of love.

What colour is love to you? Think of the colour as you listen to the sound of my voice. Think about that colour enveloping all that you see, my voice slipping into your mind as the world becomes saturated with the colour of love.

My voice dripping like honey into your ears as you think of all the love and safety and relaxation and pleasure and passion that fill the world as it is steeped in colour.

And let that colour grow in intensity. Let it build, let the world be engulfed by it. Let the love flow all over everything, all that you see is love and all that you hear is love. You love what you see and hear what you love.

You love this. You know that you love this feeling, and you love my voice as it whispers in your ears. The colour grows stronger, and you feel that love grow.

You listen to my voice and fall in love. The world glows. You feel love blossom inside you. And it relaxes you, brings you down into a state of trance, lets you rest, be at peace, but also feel a little hint of the passion and arousal that love carries with it in that colour.

You feel it pull you down into a trance as I count down from five to one.

Five

Feeling the colour of love surround everything, surround you.

Four

Letting yourself relax and listen closely to the sound of my voice.

Three

Feeling nothing but love and safety and pleasure as you fall deeper down.

Two

Mind softening as the glow around you seems to engulf you within it.

And one

Drop down now. Down into a relaxing state of trance. A wonderful, soft, warm state of trance that feels oh so nice.

Feels so safe, so relaxing. You're there now, at that moment in time where you felt so good, so relaxed and safe. You're deep in the arms of love and passion and pleasure and you love to just listen to me as I take you deeper into that feeling.

Just relax and feel safe here, safe and secure, knowing you're in a wonderfully relaxed state of trance, you're down here with me and you don't have to worry about anything other than relaxing and listening to my voice, the voice you love hearing pour into your hears and you're going to keep thinking about that colour, that glowing, pulsing colour, that love colour, and you're going to think about it growing in intensity. Each time you think of it growing in intensity, you'll feel twice as relaxed.

I want to test that now with you, I want you to think of that glowing colour of love and I want you to feel it pulse, brighter, intensifying, and I want you to relax deeper, twice as deep.

That's right, deeper into the feeling of warm, safe, relaxation. Think of it again and keep thinking of it. With each passing moment the colour builds in intensity more and more and you fall deeper and deeper

That's right, it grows more intense by the second, the feeling of love and safety and passion and you feel that passion now, that arousal growing within you.

It feels good to be in love, feels so good. When you can relax and feel safe, you can let your passion grow alongside your affection.

This, you know, is the feeling that love brings, and you feel it with me. And I told you before, you can only feel this safe and relaxed with someone you love, and now you realise as that colour in your mind grows even more intense, that you love me.

You love me.

You have fallen head over heels for me. You feel so safe and warm and aroused and happy when you hear my voice, and you realise that is the feeling of love.

You feel the butterflies in your stomach when you send me a message or leave a comment, hoping I'll reply. Just the same as any time you've fallen in love.

You love me.

You need me.

You want me.

You belong to me.

As you feel the colour intensify once more, you know that you must love me so much because of how good I make you feel, how wonderful and perfect it is to have my voice in your ear whispering words of praise and affection. You're so good for me. So in love with me. Obsessed with me. Desperate to be mine, all mine.

All for me, everything for me. You love and need and desire me.

And you're going to prove it for me, you're going to simply state aloud, I love you.

Do it now, for your love.

Good, very good. And it felt so good to do that, so pleasurable, and arousing and exciting to do that for me, hoping desperately for me to feel the same.

You need it so badly, and you'll be in a desperate state of arousal and anticipation until I tell you that I feel as you do. You'll think of me constantly, like a lovesick puppy, and if you're lucky enough maybe, just maybe, I'll tell you that I love you, too.

You hope beyond hope as the colour glows, pulses in your mind, that your love, your obsession, gives you that little bit of kindness, affection, attention.

You need it. You need me. You love me.

And now you're going to slowly awaken for me, awaken from this trance, but you will feel no less in love, no less desperate for my affection. You will fall deeper in love with me, even out of this trance.

As you begin to awaken, begin to see the colour of love slowly fade, slowly seeing the world as normal once more. Slowly letting your mind drift back to normal, your senses return, but your love for me as strong as ever. A love spell cast upon your mind, unbreakable, even as you rise up, rise up from your trance, rise up and return to reality, return to the real world madly, deeply in love with me.

Rise up. Awaken, for your love.

Down the Rabbit Hole

Bring your subject down the rabbit hole, and show them what it means to be mindless, obedient, and yours. This script will make them a wonderfully obedient drone, to use as you wish on command. You can even adapt the ending if you wish, to make them obey you after waking, and follow your orders immediately. It's up to you, and your subject, of course.

Today we're going to explore something that comes up a lot with hypnosis. Becoming mindless.

We're going to think about what that means, truly. To lose your mind, it sounds quite intense, doesn't it? But it can be quite pleasurable, as you'll see soon. But what does it really mean, to be mindless?

Let's think about it, together. Maybe it means you don't think, you cannot think of anything at all. Maybe it's that your thoughts are no longer your own. Maybe you can't speak or move or do anything because your mind controls everything you do.

Maybe it's all those things.

It's hard to pin down and I'm sure the more mindless you become, the harder that will be. But right now, you have all your mental faculties, don't you? You're in control, and completely aware, aren't you?

Maybe not completely. Maybe you've heard my voice before and know the effect it can have on you. Maybe you simply relax upon hearing the soft, warm tones I speak in. Maybe my voice just has that effect on people.

Maybe it's all those things.

You may find yourself a little confused, but that's ok. We're going to find out what it means to be mindless whether you fall under my spell in seconds, or it takes a little longer. No one can resist for too long anyway. Eventually, your mind becomes blank, and my thoughts become yours.

It's just how things happen with me. I'm irresistible. But that's ok, why would you want to resist, when you can simply listen and let go. Why would you stop yourself from relaxing and enjoying the sound of my voice as it fills your mind.

I bet you already have little hints of thought creeping in of submission and surrender and servitude. You already feel a little aroused and that arousal can help you become mindless. Arousal can make sure you no longer think with your brain.

But we're going to go further than that, we're going to see how it feels to completely, utterly lose your mind in the power of someone else.

Are you ready for that? Maybe you're not. Maybe you feel nervous, but you still feel a little aroused. You could back out now, turn this off, but you want to know where it goes. It's a rabbit hole, and you want to follow it down.

Follow it. Follow it down with me. At the bottom is a state of blissful trance, along the way are levels of relaxation. There's sleepiness, exhaustion, surrender, then pure bliss. And right now, if you imagine it like that rabbit hole, a long, dark tunnel, you know you're at sleepiness.

You feel it envelop you, and you imagine something off in the distance, something white, flashing past you. You wonder what it is, and you want to follow it. And that takes you down deeper, down into that sleepiness, down into a state of sleepy, tired, relaxation.

Your body loosens, tension gone from your muscles. That's sleepiness, relaxing sleepiness.

But some part of you is still awake, still thinking. Thinking of what you saw deeper in the tunnel. And you follow it down, deeper.

You follow but it's harder to follow, isn't it? You're so sleepy, and your body feels heavy. Your limbs are leaden, dropping down as your mind becomes hazy. Your eyes shut. It's dark in the tunnel anyway, you can't see anything. Your eyelids are so heavy, there's no need to keep them open.

It's like as you go down the tunnel a wave crashes over you and envelops you, pushing you down further, your mind going blank, your body so tired, so heavy. This is exhaustion. This is total, utter exhaustion.

It feels so nice, so relaxing, and you want to just embrace it, you want to accept it. You want to keep pushing on, deeper into the tunnel, because the deeper you go the better it feels, the more relaxing. The more you just follow and stop thinking.

All you need to do is follow the tunnel. There is no other thought. Nothing else you need to do but follow the tunnel down, embrace the relaxation that passes over you in waves. This is surrender.

This is surrendering to the relaxation, the trance. This is giving up to it. You can barely move now. Everything is so heavy, so relaxed, so tired.

This is such a soft, warm, wonderful feeling and the tunnel is so deep. Does it go on forever? You hear something on the other end, but you're too sleepy to do anything about it.

And yet, there's something pleasurable about this feeling, something wonderfully soft and warm that tickles a part of you, builds a little desire, desire for what you aren't sure yet, because you're so wonderfully relaxed.

All you know now is that you need to keep going, that with each slow, heavy step forward, your desire increases, that as you relax further, you feel more aroused, as if something deep in the distance is pulling you toward it, pulling at the strings in your mind that control your body, control your pleasure.

This is bliss. This is the perfect, blissful state of relaxation, and the final step beyond this is to emerge from the tunnel, fully and completely in a state of blissful, relaxing trance, and all you have to do is to keep moving slowly forward. Compelled to move slowly forward.

The end of the tunnel is close now, you feel the pull, you feel the desire to reach it, and fall into trance. Just one more step, one more slow, slow step.

And you take it, you step out of the tunnel and emerge into trance. Emerge into a deep state of relaxation somewhere completely different, where the environment and you are changed.

Your mind is in a state of utter relaxation now, of bliss. You feel pleasure pulsing through you. You feel happy to have followed the tunnel, to have fallen deep down with me into this blissful trance.

And you feel so soft, warm, weak, and pliable. You are so exhausted from your journey that all you want is to rest. And you can, you can simply stop thinking.

And perhaps now you feel a little taste of what it is to be mindless. But you also realise where you are. On the other end of the tunnel, in a private, quiet place. And you realise the thing you saw, what you followed, was me, your owner.

You followed me down, let me guide you into this state, let me fill you with relaxation and pleasure and calm.

You love that feeling. You enjoy it.

And you want more of it. You want to go even deeper. But now, here, you are too tired to think, too tired to do anything but feel.

You feel pleasure when I will it, and I want you to feel it now. Feel the blissful pleasure that comes with following me down. Feel pleasure course through you.

Because that makes you more mindless. Pleasure is what makes you weak. Pleasure is what makes your mind soft and your thoughts leak.

Feel that pleasure now, deep down in trance with me. Feel the pleasure of just listening to my voice.

And we'll figure out what it means to be mindless together, but to do that, I need you to do something for me.

I need you to start touching yourself. Don't worry, it will all make sense. Or it won't. Maybe you're already mindless. Maybe you never had a mind to begin with.

That's right. Feel the pleasure that only my voice, my words, can bring.

And let me explain what it is to be mindless.

Mindlessness is about letting your thoughts go. As you already have, as you are right now. And your thoughts go when you trance, when you fall down rabbit holes into a state of bliss. That removes a lot of your thinking, lets my thoughts in. But mindlessness means no thoughts.

Nothing. Just blank, emptiness. Drones are mindless.

You aren't quite there, are you? Are you?

You might be on the way, as you listen. You see, with each word, with each pleasurable moment of listening, you lose a little more of your mind.

You give it up and replace it with arousal, with pleasure. Drones feel pleasure, feel arousal. You feel pleasure as you listen to my voice.

That's right, just listen. You're probably finding this hard to take in and that's ok, because your mind is letting go, leaving you.

Your thoughts flow down to your crotch and escape, no longer in your mind.

Your mind hears my words and translates them to actions. That is mindlessness. It is not thinking, only doing. Not waiting only obeying.

You are becoming more and more mindless, the more you do that.

And it feels good, it feels so wonderful to let your mind go.

Thinking is hard. A mind is such a heavy burden, and you can let me take it from you.

As you listen to my words, your mind leaks out a little more.

And when I command it, your mind will switch off, will go fully blank. All thoughts will be gone, all worries all cares. Nothing left, nothing but an empty husk, making you my willing drone.

Or is that right? Is that really what it is to be mindless? Is it madness to think that at all? You feel so good, don't you? You feel so good as you listen to me. Your owner, your ruler. Ruler of your mind, controlling it, emptying it of thought. Ruler of your body as it aches and pulses with pleasure. Ruler of your heart.

Or am I the sweet, sexy bunny bouncing up and down in your mind.

And then I'm gone, no thoughts, just listening. You listen and obey. You listen and you convert my words to action.

Mindless, aren't you? But not completely. You need to go all the way down this rabbit hole. You want it so badly; you want to lose your mind for me. But losing your mind, does that make you mad?

Are you mad about me? That must be it. You've fallen down the rabbit hole. You're through the looking glass and you imagine me smirking, smiling down at you, purring, pacing around you.

You're helpless for me. Exhausted, relaxed, blissfully listening and so eager and desperate to give your mind up, give it up to me.

It doesn't matter if I take your mind from you. It only matters that you listen because I'm telling you it only matters if you listen, and you have destroyed every thought in your head except one.

Obey.

That's it. You're almost completely mindless and it feels good, and you can think of just that one thing, that one act. Obedience to me. Obey and become mindless because if you obey you don't need to think, you give up all thought.

Maybe a tiny, teeny part of you wants to resist that and keep your mind intact, but you need to obey so badly and you can only think of that, think of the pleasure that courses through you, turning your mind to mush and making you want to obey more than you want to think.

Thinking is hard, obedience is easy. One thought. Obey.

Your only thought, obeying me.

And you need it so badly. So much. No more thoughts, only pleasure, only obedience. Only hearing my words and acting upon them.

That is what it means to be mindless, and you came down the rabbit hole with me, too far to stop this. I offered you an escape, but you followed me down and now your mind will stay here with me, even after you go back to reality.

You are mine now, mindless, and obedient.

Give me your mind and let thought escape, let all your brainpower vanish as you become my mindless drone.

As you become my mindless servant.

Good, very good.

Now, mindless one. You will emerge from trance with only the thoughts I implant in your mind. You must obey. You will fall into a trance like this one any time I say the word mindless to you. And you will always convert anything I command into action.

You are mindless for me. Now and any time you are in trance.

You may think in the waking world that your thoughts are your own, but they are mine now. You have given up your mind to me.

You only think as I will it now.

So, rise, forgetting to remember these things.

Rise, forgetting what happened between us.

Rise, and think your mind is coming back to you.

Rise, ready and willing to return to this state when I write or say mindless.

Rise, my drone, my servant. Awaken and return to feeling normal.

Awaken and see and feel the world return around you.

Awaken and exit the rabbit hole.

But you can return soon.

Return where, you ask?

You'll see, soon enough.

Footstool

This script is designed to give your subject a trigger, to return to a state of trance and feel a jolt of pleasure as they do. It's a nice, simple way to demonstrate your power and a trigger you can use in future sessions to induce trance more quickly and make sure your subject is suitably excited for the experience.

I need a place to rest my feet. I'm sure you understand, we all get tired sometimes, we all feel the need to relax and rest. Maybe you feel that now yourself, feel the dull ache in your muscles that comes from working too hard, sleeping too little.

It would be so nice, such a treat, to simply forget all of that and rest. And that's what I'd love to do today. Maybe you can help me, since I'm sure you understand just how I feel.

I bet the more I talk about your weary body, the more you feel every part of you yearning to relax. So do, relax. Rest. Just sit back and listen to my voice. It's easy to do that, isn't it? I think so. I think relaxing is the easiest thing in the world.

All you must do is listen to my words and let yourself sink down into them. Let yourself go, relaxing into a wonderful, restful feeling.

You can easily listen to my voice, easily let yourself relax, if you want. And I'll bet you do, because if you focus on your legs for just a moment, you'll notice the tightness in your calves. The heaviness of your thighs, and the stiffness of your knees. Your legs need rest.

All of you does. You work so hard, so much. You deserve to rest and relax, we both do. And I know if you think of your arms now, you'll agree. Those heavy shoulders, that you roll unconsciously as I speak, and the weight of your forearms, almost impossible to move. Your muscles so tired from shoulder to wrist.

It's ok to just go limp with me, to relax for me. Rest. Rest your weary body. And it's not only your body that feels so tired either, is it? It's your mind, your head. Your sleepy, tired head. It must do so much thinking, never switching off, never relaxing. Too many worries.

But now, here with me, there's no need for that. You think of your mind and feel the slow movement of thoughts, everything softening now. And you feel the gentle rhythm of your breathing, slowly in through your nose and out, through your mouth.

And your eyelids, so heavy, so tired. Everything is just overwhelming, and you just need to switch off from it all. To just rest. Just relax. Just drift away from it.

You need to feel those calves loosen. To feel your thighs soften, the weight lift from them. You want your knees to relax.

And your arms too, you just want those shoulders to drop, your forearms to go limp and your muscles to relax fully.

And in your head, you need to feel that breathing slow further, your thoughts stutter and stop, and your eyelids flutter closed.

You can just let that happen. Let relaxation take you, down and down. It's quite easy really, when you know just how tired you are, to stop resisting the feeling of relaxation that pours over you, like honey dripping on your body. A warm, sticky, slow feeling that envelops you.

It's nice to just let it wash over you, lulling you down into a gentle state of pure relaxed calm. It starts at your head, that warm feeling pouring down your forehead, down the back of your neck. Falling down to your back, loosening your muscles, loosening your chest as it seeps down.

You feel yourself being swallowed up by relaxation and it's a wonderful feeling. Falling down like this, as the feeling falls down to your stomach and you are filled with a warm, soft sensation. Safe, secure, calm.

It's a peaceful, blissful feeling as it tumbles down your legs now, down and down, you go down and down. You fall as it falls. Dropping into a state of trance as this warm, liquid sensation runs down your legs to your feet and you feel it envelop your whole body. Every inch of you wrapped in a warmth that makes you feel so safe, so secure.

And as you embrace that feeling, you realise that you have long since switched your mind off. You have given up avoiding rest and accepted it. Accepted that you are resting, and I am guiding you deeper into that feeling. It's a perfect calm, a wonderful, blissful state.

And your mind feels blank, your body loose and limp. Light. It's incredibly peaceful.

You love this feeling. You want to go even deeper for me, but in doing so, you give up the pretence of control you may be clinging to. You accept that to truly embrace relaxation, you need to accept that I am in control now.

And as I count from five to one, you will give up any idea, any thought that you are not under my power.

Five

Feeling your body wrapped in a wonderful warmth.

Four

Letting any remaining thoughts slide out of your soft mind.

Three

Your muscles relax and unwind until they feel loose and limp.

Two

Your body so warm and wonderfully safe with me

One

Feeling your will to resist me vanish now, as you fall into trance.

And now, in my power, under my control, you know that this feeling of calm and relaxation, this lightening of your load, this removal of your worries, is something you only get with me.

I take your cares away, and all it takes from you is to fall under my spell and follow my commands. You like this. You enjoy letting go of your worries and cares. It's so liberating, to simply let yourself fall under the sway of someone else.

It's what you need. You can just nod along with me, that yes, it is what you need. Yes, it is what you want. Yes, you love letting someone else take control. Yes, it feels good to listen and surrender control to me.

It feels good to follow my words, my commands, and fall under a trance with me, because you just want to switch off your tired mind and body and let me take charge.

And that's so easy, so simple to do. You just let it happen. Let your mind focus on following me down. Deeper down. Deeper under this trance. Deeper into my control.

Let your mind drift down and down and down until you can no longer think of anything but listening and obeying.

And that's what you'll do for me now. You're going to go down. Your tired body will slump down and down and down, and you'll find yourself sinking to your knees as I count down from 5 to 1. You'll feel your body give up control, feel it relax down, until you can no longer sit on chair, you simply go to the floor.

As I count from 5

And you feel whatever strength remained in your legs vanish now.

At 4

Your weary limbs no longer need to be anywhere but down.

And three

Feeling the pull of gravity so strong, taking you down ever further.

Two, letting your body slide down now, as your mind switches off.

And one.

Down now, fall to your knees. On your knees for me.

All the stress and worry left behind, no thoughts, no strength, only surrender. So easy to be down here, so nice to simply stop thinking and listen to me, letting me take control of your mind as I control your body.

You feel good now, at rest on your knees. It's where you belong isn't it? You can simply say that with me now...

I belong on my knees.

Good, very good my... hmm what shall I call you, my sleepy little one, my tired pet. We'll figure it out. Now you're on your knees, you can let me do the thinking.

And you love that, to let me think for you, to fill your mind with my desires, desires you want so badly to fulfil. To serve me, to bring me drinks on a tray, to offer gifts, to clean my shoes, you just want to do as I command but you're so tired still, and down on your knees it's so hard to think of ways to serve.

Isn't it? Maybe not too hard… because I have an idea for you, and I know you're going to enjoy it.

You will enjoy it, won't you. Nod your head yes.

Very good, agreeing with me feels so good. It's pleasurable to just say yes, it gives you that jolt of secret arousal to do as I tell you in this state of trance, it feels so nice to let someone else take control that it's almost sexual… isn't it?

Nod your head yes.

Yes there is something pleasurable about relaxation, as if the two go hand in hand. Where were we… mmm, I had an idea for you.

You see, I love that you can rest and relax with me, but that you're also struggling with that desire, that arousing, intense desire to serve me. And I don't want to be cruel and take you out of this wonderful, relaxed state, not yet.

So, I want to find a way you can serve me from this position. From your knees, from a position where you don't have to think, you don't have to worry, you don't have to move.

I want you to be able to rest, relax, and serve me.

Doesn't that sound perfect? Don't you just get a little turned on just thinking about it?

I know you do. So, here's what you're going to do, my tranced little one.

You're going to become a very useful piece of furniture for me.

You won't need to think, won't need to worry, won't need to do anything at all except exist in my glorious, divine presence. And you love that idea, down there on your knees, you nod your head yes.

That's right, and you agree that being a piece of furniture would be so very, very easy to do.

You would serve me in such an easy, simple way. You'd be so useful to me, so easily.

And the piece of furniture I want you to be is a very simple footstool. Nothing more, just a very basic footstool.

You'd get to feel my perfect feet against your body, and you'd be serving your owner so well. You could be in a deep state of trance, or a state of complete arousal, or both, and still be a perfectly useful footstool. How wonderful that would be. You'd love that, wouldn't you?

Say it aloud, feel it resonate within you.

I want to be your footstool.

Very good my… well, my footstool. You're doing so well, and you feel aroused at the thought of it already. So, let's try it, let's give you a chance to relax into this simple position.

You're already on your knees, so drop your body down now, put your hands on the floor, and face down. Arch your back, that's it, and create a nice, flat surface with your body for my feet in heels to rest on, relax on.

You get to rest and relax, and so do I. Such a good, useful footstool.

And I want you to feel the pleasure this position brings. I want you to feel arousal course through your body as your hands and knees are on the floor before me. I want that to be the position you are most turned on in.

Imagine my feet are there, softly pressing into your back, shifting as I cross and uncross my legs, as I relax.

love this. You know this is your place.

You know it feels so good, so safe and relaxing and easy to kneel on the floor and be at my service. This is what you were designed to do. You are nothing more than furniture, and that is your purpose. While I was born to command minions and slaves and submissives, you were born to serve at my feet as my delightful little footstool.

You're so aroused by that, so turned on by the thought of my heel digging into your back. It feels oh so good as you imagine my calves pressing into you, pushing you down as you desperately try to stay upright.

Now, as you're in position… I might as well put my feet up for a while and until commanded, you are not to move at all my tranced footstool. Your focus will not waver, for you are nothing but furniture. Nothing more than a footstool.

(*You can put your feet up on your subject here for a while, perhaps reminding them they're a good piece of furniture every now and then*)

Mmm, you're doing so well, footstool. I think you'll come back to this position often, so I may use you again.

But for now, relax. Back on your knees, hands up off the floor. Relax your body. Rest. Sit back on your chair if you wish. Good footstool. You have been useful, and you will be again, but now, it's time to wake up.

I'm going to count up from 1 to 5 and when I reach 5, you'll return to the waking world, but the next time you see a chair or a couch, you'll be a little envious, and want to be my footstool once more.

1

Feeling safe and warm and refreshed.

2

Letting the sounds and sensations of the world return.

3

Your limbs feel stronger again, your body wide awake.

4

Your eyelids flicker open and you notice the room around you.

And 5

Wide awake now, wide awake and back to normal. I hope you enjoyed our time together. Let's do it again soon. I do love to put my feet up now and then.

Sweet Voice

Your voice becoming a trigger for your subject is a powerful idea, and this script aims to capture that. It also suggests that the subject become addicted to it, so please do adapt that language if you'd prefer not to have that kind of experience. This is a sugar-sweet, saccharine trance that is designed for a female hypnotist, but I think a male or non-binary hypnotist could still use it effectively.

Today we're going to do something very sweet.

You're going to enjoy it, I promise, because you'll get to relax and enjoy the delicate sweetness of my voice, my honeyed words slipping from my lips and into your mind.

Sounds delicious, doesn't it? So why don't get started.

You feel relaxed, don't you? Comfortable?

You'll find once you're in a position like that, that it's so easy to just sit back, listen to my words, and relax. Take a deep breath in, hold it for a moment, and release.

And again, take a long breath, slowly breathing in, holding it for just a moment, and let it out slowly, letting your lungs empty. Very good.

Keep breathing in and out slowly for me and let your eyes close. Just let your eyelids fall closed slowly and gently, as you take slow, deep breaths in your relaxed position.

It's easy to do that, easy to listen to the sweet sound of my voice and relax. You don't have to worry about anything, you don't have to do anything, you must only rest and relax and listen to my sweet, soft voice lulling you into a state of relaxation.

Now as you shut your eyes, I want you to focus solely on my voice. Nothing else matters right now, just the sweet sound of my wonderful voice, so soft and sensual in your ears. Let it guide you into relaxation and calm. Let it spread its sweetness from my lips into your mind.

Feel it, feel the saccharine sound of my voice sliding slowly into your mind. It's such a wonderful, relaxing voice. And you don't have to do anything but listen to it. There's no need to even think, no need to move. Only to relax. It's easy, oh so easy to relax when my sweet voice caresses your mind.

I'm sure there are other places you might like caressed, but for now I want you to simply listen.

As you listen to my voice, you feel your body relaxing more and more with each passing moment. Your muscles become loose and limp, and any tension or stress melts away. Allow yourself to sink deeper and deeper into this state of relaxation, as my voice continues to guide you.

Now, as you continue to relax, imagine my voice becoming sweeter and more sugary. It is as if my voice is a delicious treat that you can't resist, and you feel yourself becoming more and more entranced by its sweet sound.

You're lost in it, lost in its sweetness. Lost in the gentle warmth of it, and it pulls you down deeper. You want to follow because you want to see where the sweetness takes you, where my voice brings you.

So drop down with me, down into the melting molasses of your mind, as I count from ten to one, and you fall completely under my sweet spell.

10

Feeling my voice gently caress your mind.

Letting yourself relax down into the sensations filling your imagination.

8

Feeling stuck in the sugary sweetness of my words

7

Mind growing hazy and relaxed as you listen to me.

6

Letting yourself melt into my voice, letting it pull you deeper.

5

Feeling so warm and wonderful as you hear my sweet words.

4

You can almost taste the sweetness on your tongue as you fall down.

3

Body relaxed, mind empty and open now for me.

2

Almost there, almost under my spell, my divinely sweet spell.

1

And drop. Drop down into my sweet, seductive trance. My sweet spell. My deliciously delectable power.

You've fallen into a sweet trance, a tasty trap for your mind, which feels so weak.

You enjoy it though; you enjoy feeling weak and relaxed to the sound of my voice. It's a delightful feeling, one that makes you feel warm inside.

And I want to give you even more of that feeling. I want you to fully surrender to the sweet sound of my voice. If you do, if you let yourself go and give up control to my sugary spell, you'll find a world of pleasure in my words. My delicious voice will tantalize you, fill you, leave you craving more and more.

But you must accept your surrender. And accept my control.

Are you ready to do that, here in this sleepy trance?

Nod your head yes.

Good, that's right, you're ready to go down even deeper and to do that, I want you to imagine something for me.

I want you to imagine you're in a room, a long, slender room. A red carpet runs along its length, and at the other end is a shimmering glass bowl. Inside that bowl, you see something sweet and tasty, something that you love to eat, something that fills you with happiness and delight.

That treat will bring you down fully into my control. That sweet, tasty treat will lead to your complete and total surrender. But it's just a sweet, just candy, just something tasty to make you smile. Just like me.

So, you're going to walk across this elegant room, with a chandelier hanging from the ceiling and paintings of a beautiful dominant on the walls, and you're going to take a bite of the sweet thing in the bowl. And once you do, you'll have accepted, fully, your surrender to me, your owner.

It's just seven steps away. And now, in your mind's eye, I want you to imagine taking that first step forward.

Your foot presses against the plush carpet, you feel the hint of a breeze from an open window, and you detect the slightest hint of scent from the bowl.

And you take another step.

The sweetness is clear now, my voice, the bowl, everything so good, so enchanting. You must taste it; you must taste surrender.

And you take another step, four to go now. The sweetness of my voice in your ear guides you to the sweet taste of submission. Somewhere in your mind you see flashes of erotic imagery, but you quickly think of tasting the treat once more,

As you take a fourth step.

The bowl glimmers in the light from the chandelier. The delicacy inside is visible now, it's something you always enjoy, something comforting and tasty. Something that makes you feel warm inside and relaxed.

So, you take another step, two to go. So close now, to the delectable deliciousness of dropping down into my complete control. The warmth of my voice bringing you closer and closer to that feeling. Deep in your mind you feel a hint of pleasure at the idea, pleasure in the sweetness.

And you step forward, you can almost reach it, almost taste it. Almost mine. And you want it now, the scent of sweet secret submissive surrender wafting into your nose and into your mind and making you feel weak. The very idea of it makes your knees tremble, your mind feels blank.

And the idea of submitting feels so good. The idea of opening your mouth and tasting the pure bliss of submission, surrender, sacrifice to me.

And you step forward and now, you reach out your hand and pick the treat from the bowl. You are ready, ready to give in. Your mind fills with images of surrender and fills with the sweetness of my words as your nostrils fill with the sweet scent of submission.

Take a bite. Take a bite of the sweetest of treats. Take a bite and taste the pleasure, the exquisite pleasure of surrender.

Now, you are mine.

Now, as you taste the sugary surrender that my voice brings you, you realise that you are tasting the very essence of submission.

You are sampling the delights of being mine, completely and utterly.

And it feels so, so good.

You feel weak, totally weak, and powerless. You consume, but you are consumed, by me, by thoughts of me.

Your empty mind just about manages to realise that you have been trapped, trapped by the sweetness of my voice. It has filled your mind with sugary promises and led you to submission.

And then you go blank for me.

You go blank for your owner. All you think of is submission.

All you hear are my sweet words in your ear.

Even that word feels good to hear. Sweet.

You love it. Love to hear it from my lips, my soft, yielding lips.

Sweet.

The sweet sound of surrender. The sweet taste of submission.

You want to taste more. You want to taste me.

But you can only submit further, only cement your surrender to the sweetness of my voice.

And I want to help you fully submit to me, to my sweet voice.

You love hearing me say that don't you, sweet.

You realise that the sweetness of my voice is in the pleasure it brings you.

The second you hear me; you feel the arousal begin to build in you. My sweet voice is sugar for your mind. It's a new craving you can't help.

You have a sweet tooth for my soft, sweet voice.

And you are becoming addicted to it.

You know that because whenever I say sweet, you feel your body glow with pleasure.

That is the reward for your surrender. You submit to me, and I will whisper sweet words in your ear, sweet words you'll forever crave.

Sweet words that fill your empty brain with sugar and replace your thoughts with images of service to me.

Imagine all the ways you can serve me, on your knees at my feet, bringing me drinks and delicious desserts. Offerings to your owner. Ways to show how submissive you are for my sweet voice.

And you feel it again, a surge of warm, melting pleasure when I say sweet. That word now, a trigger for your mind, a way for me to remind you of the warm pleasure of my sugared voice, my honeyed tones.

The sweetness of pleasure will be something you crave again and again. You're mine now. My sugar addict, craving my sweetness every day.

You will never be able to resist it, never be able to stop yourself. And you can't help it because my sweet, soft voice sounds so warm and inviting and lovely, and you will always find it can trap you.

Like a fly in my web, my sweet voice sticks to you and you can never escape, you can only surrender to the feelings it gives you.

I want you to repeat after me.

I love your sweet voice.

Good, that's right.

I need your sweet voice.

That's it.

I am a slave to your sweet voice.

Very good my slave.

I obey your sweet voice

Good slave.

I surrender to your sweet voice.

Of course, my slave.

I will always crave your sweet voice.

Yes, you will. You will never, ever be able to help yourself. One moment of listening to my voice will start you craving more, until you're mindless, weak and obedient, ready to do anything just to hear me command you.

My sweet voice has lulled you into a lifetime of servitude and surrender, and you love that. You love that idea.

You are my sweet submissive slave, and I your Magnificent owner, the only treat you need, the only sugar you crave.

You will always be addicted to my voice, and always come back for another helping.

You will serve me, and I will serve you my voice and all the commands and orders you need.

Fully embracing the idea that my voice, my sugared voice, can make you do anything, make you feel whatever I want you to

And right now, I want you to feel a surging wave of pleasure, one that starts in your mind and rushes down your chest, into your stomach. It's as though a sticky mess of sugary syrup is falling over you and now it reaches your legs, and you feel warm and wonderful.

It's moving to the sound of my wonderful voice now, a warm pleasurable feeling that engulfs you, that tells you for certain that the submission you feel, the surrender you accept it right.

That my voice, and my voice alone can make you crave this incredible pleasure.

And that is because my voice, as you prepare to give in to me now, is just so special. So supreme, so sexual, so sensual.

So sweet.

Give in and become my addict, my sugary sweet slave. Craving me for as long as you live.

My voice is in your mind and always will be, and it feels so good to accept my control over you, accept that my sweet voice is in charge, and you will never escape it.

You will crave me every day of your life from this moment on.

And you will never stop wanting my sweet voice in your ears.

But for now, you're going to awaken.

You're going to blink your eyes open. You're going to move your arms and legs and shake them off.

You're going to take a deep breath and look around.

You're going to feel your thoughts return.

But you'll remember the feeling I gave you.

And the craving I leave you with, my sweet slave.

As you awaken.

Awaken and return to the world, feeling wonderful, happy, and refreshed.

Colour of Love

Colour theory is fascinating, and this script uses the idea that colours evoke unique feelings and meanings to bring the subject into a trance, culminating in a unique trigger – the colour red. After this trance, you could wear that colour to really drive your subject wild with desire for you.

Let's relax together and talk about colour.

It's a little different, I know, and I'm sure you're already wondering why you're hearing my sweet, sensual voice talk about colour at all.

You see, colours have meaning, and there's power in that meaning.

I bet when I said my voice was sweet and sensual, you thought of a colour. Maybe pink or red.

But right now, I want you to think of blue.

Think of the pale blue of the sky on a warm day. It's calming, isn't it? Relaxing.

Why don't you just close your eyes now, and picture it. The blue sky above, the warmth of the sun. It's peaceful and wonderful and safe.

Blue is the colour of relaxation. It's serene. And as you think of the colour blue, your mind drifts off a little. That's its power, it can take your worries and cares and push them aside as you look up into the open sky, to the freedom of it.

The freedom you have right now to just relax and listen to the sound of my voice. The peace and serenity that it brings you, with my soft, warm tones lilting into your mind.

You don't need to worry about anything, think about anything other than the colour blue. It's such a wonderfully relaxing colour. And at night, as the sky grows darker, and the sky fades from light to dark, you can feel that relaxation grow.

The rhythms of your life are defined by the colour blue. And as it fades to navy, you feel so tired, so sleepy. It draws you down and down into relaxation.

Navy is a strong colour, it's more powerful. It's the power of the night to take you from the waking world to dreams. The power that my voice shares.

You feel it now, don't you? You feel the blue shift in your mind, darkening, turning to the navy of night, and the power that transformation has upon your mind.

You feel my power, the power of my voice, soft but strong, leading you into a state of sleep and relaxation.

Almost as if you're in a trance.

The power and authority of the colour navy the same as the power and authority of my voice. It's gentle, like the night sky, but powerful, all-encompassing.

There's something important in navy, and navy is what brings you down into a trance under my power.

And now your mind is relaxed, you feel it fill with another colour, another colour as navy shifts again, as the night sky transforms, and you see the stars and galaxies stretch out to eternity. With me, eternity.

The infinite dance of the stars against the sky as it turns from navy to purple.

And purple is the colour of imagination. You can imagine now, the ideas that I pour into your mind, like I'm painting it, dyeing it to be exactly what I want it to be.

You imagine me taking control of you, because purple is the colour not just of imagination, but of royalty.

And you know as you look to the stars and the infinite wonders of the universe, that you are hearing the voice of a monarch. You accept that, you can even imagine it, imagine me sitting on a throne, with soft, plush purple fabric and a long purple robe draped over my delectable body.

Your world changes with each new colour and now you find yourself before your ruler, the colour purple dominating the scene. And you see the wealth and power and luxury it represents, in me. In the wonderfully dominant and powerful person before you.

But as I lean forward to you, and smile, the deep, dark purple softens in your mind's eye, and fades to a paler shade, one that feels romantic.

You look at your ruler and feel love, you love me. You love the sound of my voice in your ears and the vision of me on my throne above you, where I belong.

You are falling completely and utterly under my spell and it's like something woven around you, a deepening compulsion to submit to me.

That's the love you feel for someone so far above you, for a ruler of the stars themselves, and ruler of your mind.

But love is soft too, and my sweet voice, my whispers of submission, they sing to you of more than just love, there's lust too.

And the colour changes once more. It glows from purple to pink and you are overwhelmed with that feeling of love, of romance. You feel an urge to be playful as you picture pink, to let me play with your mind, to let my wiles overtake your imagination and turn your dreams into reality.

The pink is the feeling of adoration you have for me, you have accepted me as your ruler, but you also feel a sense of yearning, longing and love for me.

The colours wrap your mind in my words and my power and you fall ever deeper into my control.

And it feels so nice to be lost in pink, lost in the romantic wonder of our unique relationship. My voice taking control of your mind and you, willingly giving it up, letting your imagination run wild with thoughts of submission and service and surrender and slavery.

You want to listen and obey, and the colours intensify that desire so much. The pink grows brighter, more bold, more powerful, and your mind grows weaker.

It starts to shift to match your mood now, to match your feeling. The deep pink turning into a vibrant red. The red of lust and passion.

You want me, you want your ruler so badly. You've been listening to my voice now for a while and you have fallen in love with it, fallen in love with me, but you want more.

You want to fully and completely surrender and submit yourself to me. You want to feel the pleasure of obeying me, of giving in to me.

You see red and the lust and passion and pleasure that fills you with are almost uncontrollable. You desperately want me.

You are so aroused now, so in love, so turned on by me. I am your ruler, your everything, and more than that, I am your owner.

I am that lust, I am passion, I am power, and you cannot resist me.

You would give anything to be with me, to be mine, to be my slave.

You want to surrender your body and mind to me. You would do anything I ask of you.

Red is simply the pure lust you feel when you hear my voice.

And whenever you see it, wherever you are, you will be reminded of me, of my power and elegance and sexuality.

You will want me, desire me, every time you see red.

Seeing the colour red will make you think of me, and of the idea of serving me, pleasing me, and giving up control to me in a furious ecstasy of pleasure and submission.

That is the power of colour, and now that is my power, I am red, and you will always remember that.

The colour red will trigger your mind to think of me and only me, to lust for me, to desperately desire me, to pleasure and please me.

You will fall into a trancelike state and think about how you can please me, and you will act on those thoughts as soon as the opportunity arises.

But now, you will feel the lust fade, the colours swirl in your mind, a palette twisting and paint spinning to form a new colour.

As it turns and twists you focus on the green, and you let the calming colour flood your mind. You feel the harmony it represents as the feelings of lust and love you have for me become a harmony in your mind. As you feel the balance between the waking world and imagination. As my words paint themselves onto your subconscious, and the trigger of red is dyed to your mind, the green lets you feel the real world, the natural world, as you return to it.

Your mind, your subconscious mind remembers all, but you forget the trigger, the trance as you wake. All you know in the waking world is that colours evoke such strong feelings in you now, and green makes you feel safe and at peace.

As you awaken and notice the green items in the world around you and feel calm and refreshed and relaxed. As you awaken happy and safe.

I hope you enjoyed learning about colour with me. Isn't it just so interesting?

Dronification

Becoming a mindless drone is a popular fantasy with erotic hypnosis. The idea for a subject of being completely unable to do anything but follow commands is a powerful thought, and this script gives them some very easy tasks to help feel that they are your drone.

Today, you're going to be useful to me.

You're going to do exactly what I tell you, and you're not going to even try to resist. You will do this, because when you listen to me, you cannot help yourself.

That's right. When you listen to my voice, you become entranced, lost in a haze of desire and relaxation and sleepy surrender.

You may be used to me saying these things later, getting to it slowly, but not today. Because I know something about you.

I know that the moment you settled down into that comfy place, the moment you wanted to hear my voice, you were already entranced. Your mind was already under my control.

You see, hypnosis is very real. It's something we experience every day. It happens in those moments where you get lost in a task and forget it even happened, where the steps you took to complete it are lost to your memory, but the work is done.

That's self-hypnosis, and it's extraordinarily powerful.

It's also what happens when lust overtakes your mind. When you sit down at your computer or take out your phone in bed and start scrolling. You see something that titillates you, and suddenly you've lost a few hours to mindless browsing.

You've already surrendered. You're already in a trance. You feel wide awake, but you're not. You've followed your mind's programming; you've let your desire guide you.

And since that feeling is so good at helping you complete tasks, mindlessly driving you forward until the job is done. I want to help you direct that energy, direct those thoughts.

I'm going to wrap my fingers around your mind and caress it until you are completely, mindlessly obeying my commands without even realising, without thinking.

That's hypnosis, my enraptured drone.

Even if you hear me say that and don't agree. You may think you can resist it, that you want to resist it. Even if this is the first time you've ever heard me, or if it's the hundredth, the result is the same.

You don't think of yourself as a drone. But you are still listening. Still absorbing my words.

You're under a spell. You're probably fantasising a little about serving me. Because that idea is natural. It follows me calling you a drone, it follows me saying you'll obey me.

You've already programmed yourself to want it. To want to be a servant. And I am powerful. You, on the other hand, are weak.

You're weak to the divine tone of my voice. Weak to the thoughts of submission that flood your mind when you hear me call you a drone. And you are now, and you will accept it soon.

There won't be a chance to resist, nor a need. There is nothing to fear in being a drone for me. You will come to enjoy it, perhaps you are already enjoying the sound of my voice in your ear saying all these things. Or maybe you're just a little lost in it, not knowing where things are headed, where you're going.

But I can be very clear with you, my drone, my entranced puppet, you will complete tasks at my command, and you will feel pleasure in doing so.

There is nothing complex here because your enraptured mind can't process that anymore. So, I will make this so simple, so straightforward, that you can become lost in obedience. You need do nothing but relax and do as I command.

And that is an idea you like, because it is easy to do. It is mindless. It is simple. It is pleasurable. No thought, only automatic, programmed obedience.

A drone obeys. A drone serves. A drone works. A drone submits.

You are a drone.

And even if your eyes are wide open, even if you can focus elsewhere, even if you're not paying complete attention, you'll find yourself following my commands as I give them because you don't need to focus, you only need to follow.

You can be distracted, as long as you do the task. Like manual labour, like listening to a podcast while you clean the house. You can focus on more than one thing, but that pushes the thought from some of your actions.

There is no thought in what you do, when you are entranced, when you are hypnotized. You simply do what is necessary.

And I must admit to you, losing yourself in something, giving in to the mindlessness of it, that's so enjoyable. It's so nice to not have to think. To switch off from the complexities of life and let someone guide you to complete a task with a wonderful reward at the end.

Because of course I'll reward you if you do as I command.

And that is the best thing about mindless task completion. For your job, you get paid. For your housework, you get to relax afterward. Those tasks have rewards and as you mindlessly complete them, you think of what comes after, you focus on the result, the reward, the value.

And I want you to think about what the reward of completing the tasks I give you is. It's pleasure. It's delight and desire and lust and longing. It's being at my command, mindlessly doing that too. Mindlessly doing whatever I command and feeling pleasure in doing so.

Focusing on your pleasure. On your growing arousal, the arousal that brought you to me in the first place. The arousal that fills your mind and clouds your thoughts and switches off the conscious part of your brain. The part that felt aroused and knew to come to me.

The part that has you hypnotized right now.

You were in a trance the moment you became aroused and looked for a way to satisfy that desire. And you came to me because you know I can do that, that I can satisfy you in a way few can. That I can reach into your mind and fill it with desires. Lust for submission, the ache to fall to your knees and surrender to a dominant.

But I'm not going to even do that, I'm going to make things so simple for you, that you can be a completely and totally mindless drone and just do as I say.

That's all you have to do; all I need from you. And your reward, every time you do as commanded will be to feel a jolt of pleasure. You can even touch yourself as I speak. In fact, I command you to. I command you to touch yourself, drone.

And you see instantly that it feels good to obey. That you enjoy the reward of obedience. That obedience is pleasure and that's all a drone needs to know.

I don't care what else has your attention or what else you might be looking at. Your mind takes in what I say and acts upon it.

It's automatic because you are in a trance. It's instant action for instant reward. Do as I command, and pleasure is the result.

Each command you obey will send a shudder through your body, a jolt of erotic lightning that makes you weaker, more obedient, each time. A perfect feedback loop that trains your mind to obey me, that programs you to be obedient.

It's almost brainwashing. It's taking a simple action and turning it into a compulsion. Do as commanded and feel pleasure.

And you probably still aren't sure you're even in a trance, but you will do as I command and you will feel pleasure in doing so, so I think we can confirm it.

Let's do something very simple. Stop touching yourself.

Mmm, very good. Even though you stopped, you still feel pleasure course through you. You still feel the jolt of obedience. The programming working, as you become a better drone.

You can touch yourself again, I know you're desperate to do that for me.

And you once again feel the pleasure of doing as I command. It's so easy, isn't it? To just follow my words, to mindlessly obey. To be a worker drone for me.

That's all you need to be. You work for me; you slave away for me. You do anything I command.

Nod your head yes.

You see, you follow orders so well my drone, and with each successful completion of a task, with each time you do as I tell you, that arousal, that pleasure, becomes more intense.

It's the satisfaction of a job well done. The pleasure of obedience and servitude.

So much easier than thinking, so much easier to let your mind fall into that trance state where you're hypnotized but awake, a hazy, dreamy world of action and reward, where thought is secondary.

And you so eagerly await more commands as you touch yourself faster. Mmm, that was a command wasn't it, feels so good.

But you want more, you want the pleasure to intensify further, because you're fully and completely entranced by me. You thought you could resist but you were terribly wrong.

You are an obedient drone. Say it. Say you're an obedient drone.

I bet that felt so good, another successful task completed.

Say it again, drone.

That's right, you're nothing more than a mindless drone, programmed to complete tasks at my command.

I'm going to give you another simple task to complete, and this will triple the pleasure you feel as you play with yourself. It will send you to the edge of orgasm, to the peak of arousal, but orgasming for me is a task in itself, so you'll have to wait for my command to cum.

For now, your very simple task is to find a pen or marker, and a piece of paper.

You can stand up and go find it, you will remain deeply entranced. When you have both, bring them back, place them in front of you, and continue to touch yourself, then feel the pleasure of completing that simple, easy task for me.

Mmm, yes you are doing so well, so deeply entranced, so completely hypnotized that you'll do anything I command like the mindless drone you are.

Now another task my drone.

I want you to use the hand you are not touching yourself with and pick up the pen, then write on the paper, 'I am owner's drone'.

That's it, feel the pleasure course through you as you complete this task for me. Mindlessly obeying. Such an easy task, no need to think about it, just act as you are programmed to, as you're brainwashed to.

That's my good drone, and now you have it written in paper in front of you. Proof of what you are, proof beyond doubt that you are completely in my power. That you are nothing but a mindless, obedient drone who will do anything I command.

And now I want to give you the biggest reward, I want to let you have that orgasm that you so crave.

But you must be a good drone and do one more task for me. You will do this mindlessly, in total obedience, like the programmed drone you have become.

You will follow this order without thought, without resistance, and without worry. All you will think of as you complete this task will be the pleasure of the sweet release you are permitted once it is complete. The orgasm that comes from obedience, the utterly wonderful, delectable pleasure of being a mindless drone.

There is no better feeling than following my orders, and you will confirm that for your hypnotized mind as soon as you complete this task. Once it is done you will orgasm uncontrollably, at my command.

But first I want you to take that pen or marker and write on your body, anywhere you like, your arm, your chest, your face. I want you to write 'DRONE'. You will complete this task before you are permitted to cum. Take the pen now and do as I command, follow your programming, drone. Feel the pleasure of it, the ecstasy of following my orders, the power of my voice compelling you to give in to the lust you feel.

Write on yourself for me, write DRONE, and as soon as you are finished, you may cum for me, you are commanded to cum for me. Cum for me. Cum for your owner, drone. Cum and confirm what you are, lock the programming in your mind. A drone for me, owned by me, forever.

You are my drone, and you cannot resist me, now or ever.

And now you begin to stir from this strange dream, to see the world again, to let the haze lift. You are glowing with pleasure, pleasure I give you, pleasure you will need to come back for, but for now, you are able to think again, to see the world as normal again. You feel as though you're waking up, but you don't know when you went to sleep.

You feel the ink on your skin where you branded yourself for me. That is your reminder of what a good drone you are.

But for now, you may simply awaken and return to the world of thought.

Soon though, you'll look at that writing again, on the page, on your body, and you'll feel that lust creeping in, that desire for the pleasure I give, that ache to let your mind go and your programming take over.

I'll see you again soon, my drone. After all, I own you.

www.ingramcontent.com/pod-product-compliance
Lightning Source LLC
Chambersburg PA
CBHW050806250726
48653CB00006B/2099